I0838016

"To Josefina, who inspired me to write this book".

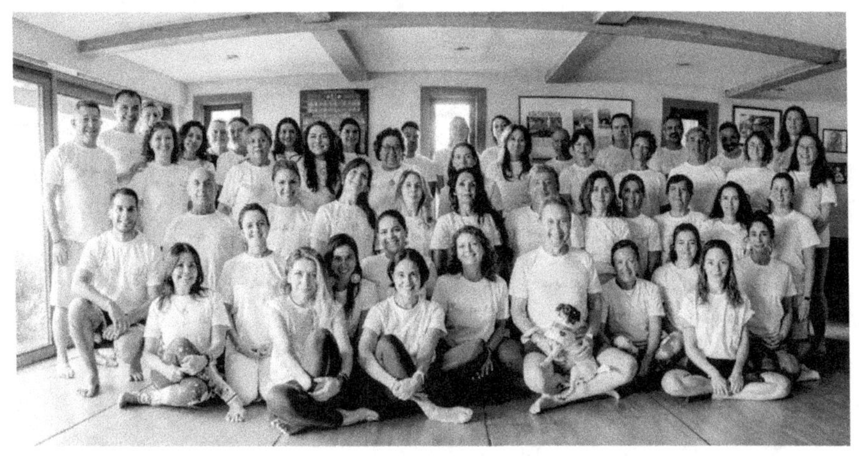

January 6th, 2024

Yoga for Life!

"The Ultimate Yoga Method"

By Gustavo Ponce

First Edition

The partial or total reproduction of this work, by any means, without prior written permission of the copyright holders is prohibited.

Photographers: Emmanuel Diaz and Alejandro Cifuentes

Design & production

Patricio Castillo Romero www.entremedios.cl

Edited in Chile

Contents

PRESENTATION

Hello! I ´am Gustavo Ponce, born in Chile in 1947. I have just hit the ripe age of 77. As I begin writing this book, it´s disheartening to observe the ongoing conflicts between Russia-Ukraine, Israel-Hamas, and others around the world where they seek to annihilate each other, and to witness the suffering of thousands escaping these confrontations. I can´t help but connect global turbulences with the internal conflicts we often experience as human beings. Yoga, is a profound discipline and philosophy that strives for the opposite of war and conflict. It seeks to unite us, starting with self-unity.

That´s why, at this historical moment, I´m excited to share with you my new approach, "Yoga for Life."

If you think of yoga just as a form of exercising your body and quietening your mind, is already a big thing. To me is much more, is a life philosophy! As exercise, and as any form of mild exercise, you probably know deep in your heart, that exercise protects your body from diseases, from old age problems and dysfunctions, and keep you in good shape to face the years ahead. On top of that, it helps you sleep well, and your work becomes more productive because it sharpens your brain. You will be in good spirits and the risk of developing chronic diseases will diminish. It is a great therapy. In fact, it amazes me that when you go to see a doctor, normally he/she takes your pulse, blood pressure, listen to your lungs and in some cases, check your body temperature. In my opinion, the doctor should also add a simple question, "how much time do you dedicate every day to do exercises?" The least we can do to be out of the reach of the radar of doctors is to walk no less than five kilometers a day. It should not take longer than 20-30 minutes. This is an aerobic exercise.

So, this method is address to everyone interested in doing a favor to their bodies and mind, but are too lazy or don´t have the motivation to do what they know they have to do. No need to go to a yoga school! You can practice at home with this book and the video. To practice Yoga for Life, all you need is a chair and 45 minutes (better one hour) of your day. Regardless of age, physical condition or sex, this method is designed for busy folks like you! In just two months, you´ll establish a daily routine that can stick with you for a lifetime.

Perfect for a morning routine, it includes a delightful blend of activities. You´ll enjoy invigorating warm-up calisthenics, rejuvenating breathwork, and strengthening exercises for arms, legs, and core. The practice not also promotes joint health, but also focuses on your internal organs, glands, hormonal balance, lymphatic channels cleansing, and on top of that, centers your mind.

You will trigger the release of "Happy Hormones" - dopamine, serotonin, oxytocin, and endorphins. Together, they team up to boost your mood and overall well-being. During exercise, especially the endorphins are unleashed, creating a sense of "Euphoria". That´s why, after a session of Yoga for Life, we feel happier and more relaxed.

Feel free to follow my video instruction or use the guidance provided in this book. Enjoy your practice, and don't give up before two months are behind you and consider it a lifelong commitment for lasting well-being! If one hour seems too much, trim it down to 45 minutes or half an hour. But remember no less! Persistence is key. Enjoy your journey to a healthier you!

Oh, and here´s something important: Don´t worry about the many techniques and poses. Some only take a few seconds, and others just a couple of minutes. Having a variety is crucial to achieving the awesome results I promised the method would bring to you.

Caution: While Yoga for Life is suitable for everybody, if you have a discopathy or any spine issues, it can still be beneficial, but is crucial to start with care. Practice the exercises mindfully and avoid excessive repetitions initially. Gradually, you can increase the repetitions as you progress.

FIRST SECTION "WAKING UP"

For an optimal Yoga for Life experience, it´s recommended to incorporate "Kechari Mudra" by pressing the tongue against the soft palate and engaging the pelvic floor as needed. Staying mindful of this muscle is key. The GPBALANCE method, detailed in www.gpbalance.com, provides ample information on the significance of these practices.

As we explore the techniques and poses of Yoga for Life, let´s delve into the importance of rewiring our brains to establish the habit of daily practice. According to Dr. Loretta Breuning, a neuroscientist and expert in science and behavior, forming a new habit can take anywhere from 21 to 90 days, varying from person to person. Developing a habit is a gradual process that relies on consistent repetition and positive reinforcement. Emphasizing the quality of repetitions and the sustainability of the behavior is more beneficial than strictly adhering to a specific time frame.

If you are tall or if your chair is not sturdy enough, I recommend doing this section using a table or something you can hold on for better stability.

17

1. ALTERNATE LEG LIFT (25 Reps with each leg)

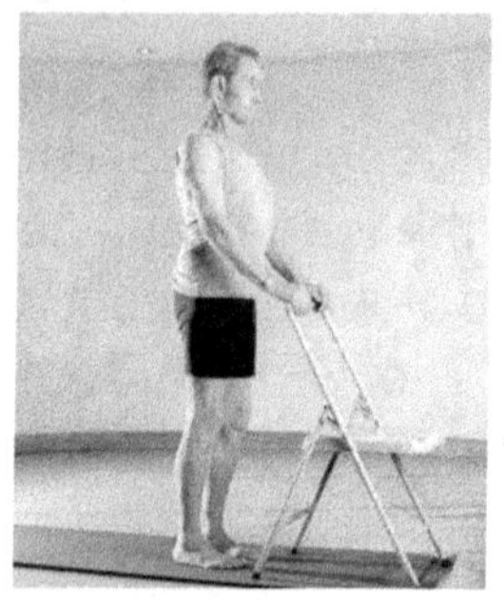 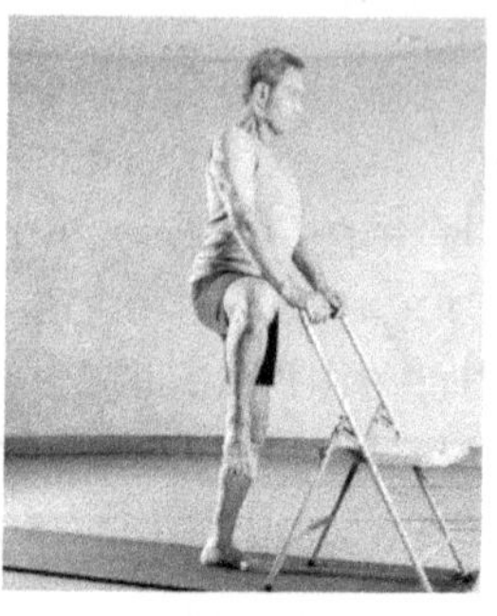 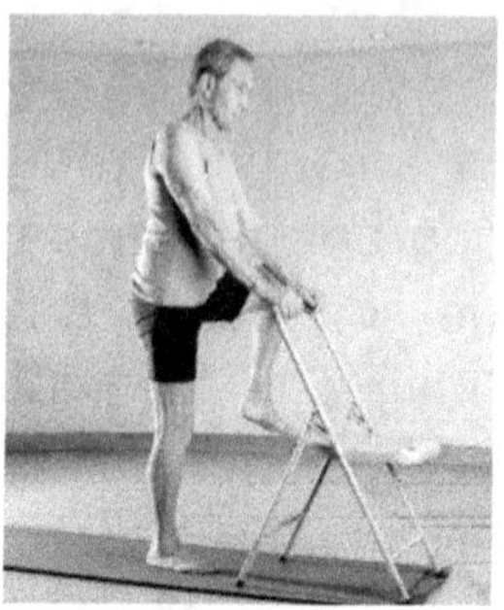

Getting into exercise mode right after waking up isn´t always the most exciting idea. So, let´s trick our minds with something super simple. Just stand up, place your hands on the back of the chair, or on a table, and start lifting your legs while you yawn. It is a gentle way to wake up your body!

2. HEEL TAPPING (10 Reps)

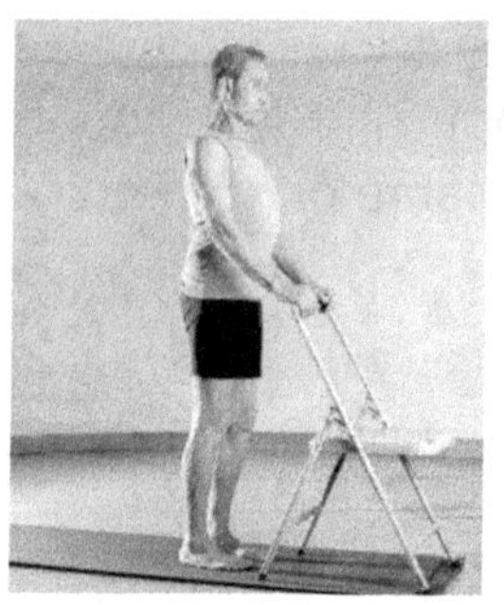 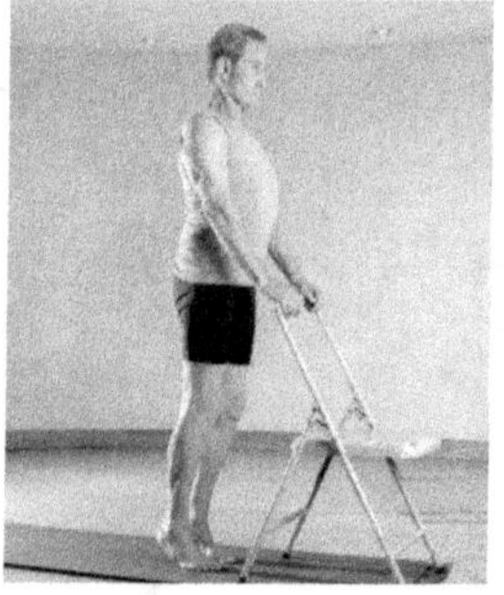 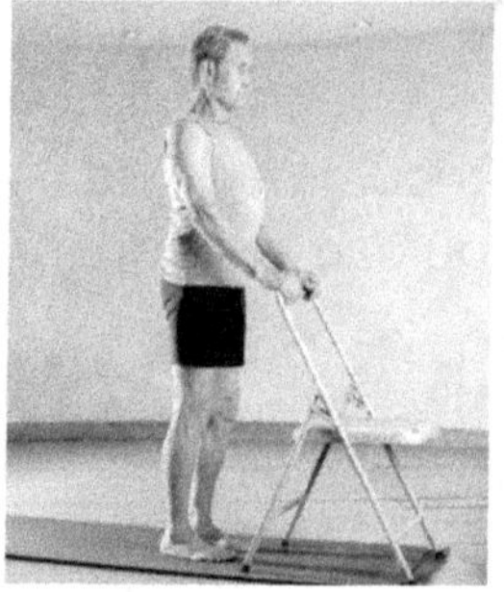

Understanding energy work, as explained by Eastern masters, can be challenging. It´s helpful to listen to their wisdom, bearing in mind that some teaching may be metaphorical. For instance, consider Mantak Chia, a Taoist teacher known for his qigong and internal alchemy. He suggests that our bodies have positive and negative poles based on the Taoist philosophy of yin and yang. According to Chia, women´s positive pole is in the head, negative in the genitals, and vice versa for men, to complement each other.

In Taoist philosophy, yin and yang symbolize interconnected and interdependent complementary forces, describing the harmony of opposite forces in existence. However, in the Western world, the idea of distinct positive and negative poles, especially associated with gender-specific anatomical areas, may not align with our understanding of human physiology.

Consider the practice of tapping a homeopathic remedy, known as "succussion". While believed to enhance the remedy, it´s essential to note that the scientific basis for this isn´t widely supported.

In the sequence of exercises, tapping the heels is believed to energize the body and reduce yawning. It´s a simple way to invigorate yourself!

3. LEGS SIDE LIFTING (10 Reps with each leg)

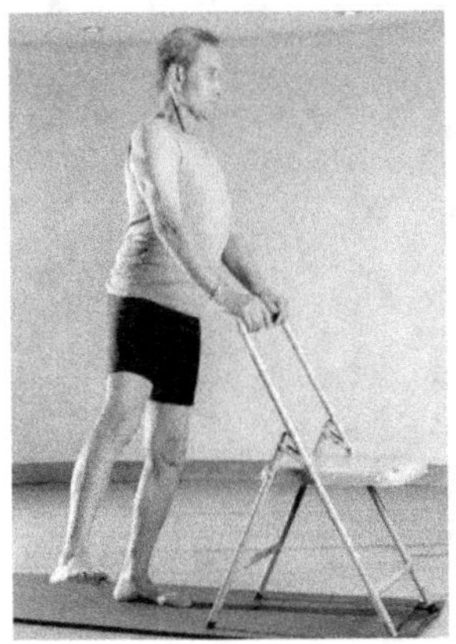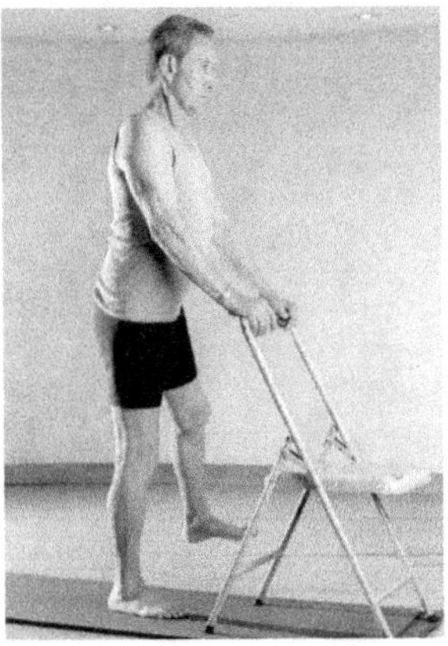

When you lift one leg, then the other, sideways while standing, it mainly engages the hip muscles. The key players in this action are the abductors, the gluteus medius and gluteus minimus, the sartorious and the hip adductors.

Coordination among these muscles is crucial for stability and controlled motion during this movement. Also, your core muscles may pitch in to maintain and support your spine while lifting the leg.

4. LEGS SIDE SWING (10 Reps with each leg)

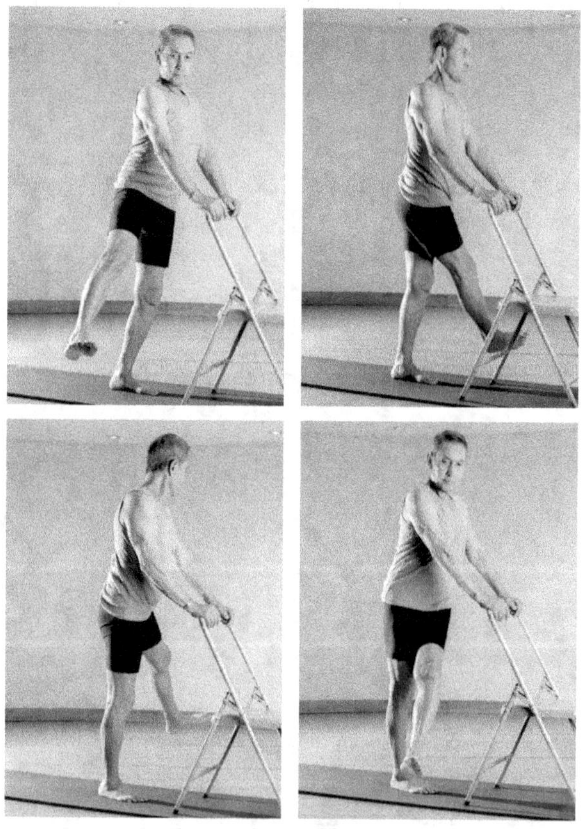

Swinging your leg side to side while standing and holding onto the back of a chair works different muscles groups to control the movement. Also, turning your head towards the leg you swing engages neck muscles. The main muscles involved are hip flexors, abductors, quadriceps, hamstrings, core, and calf muscles. Neck rotators, flexors, are also part of the action.

It Is important to do these movements smoothly and comfortably to avoid strain or injury. Stretching and strengthening exercises for these muscles can improve flexibility and stability.

5. WARRIOR 3 (10 Reps with each leg)

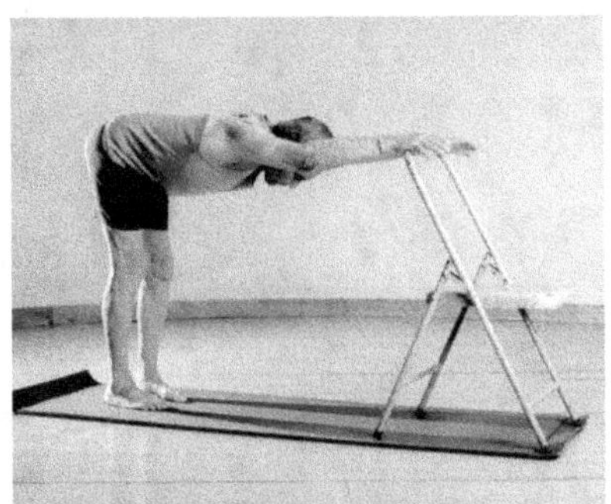
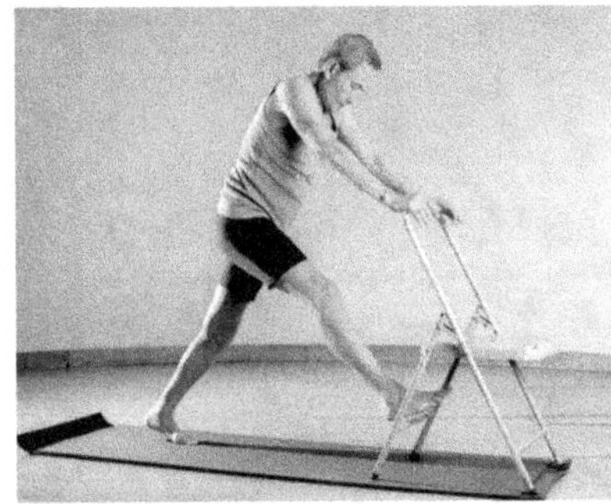

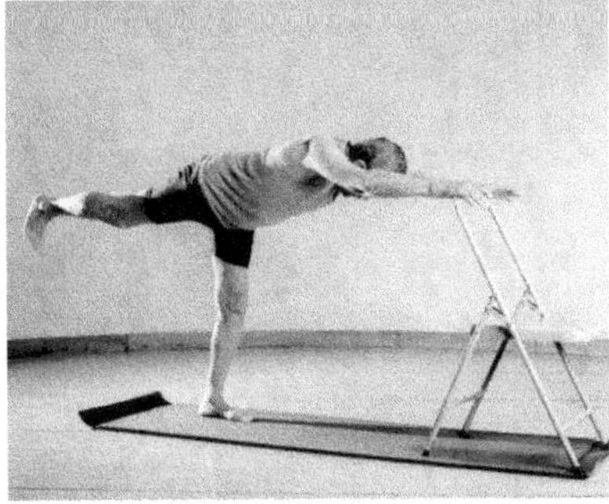

Just like with any yoga pose, it´s important to listen to your body and stay aware. This standing pose involves balancing on one leg while extending the other leg straight back, aiming for a line from your head to the heel. In Yoga for Life, we use a chair or a table for balance, making it easier to hold the posture.

Here´s how we do it: Stand with a straight body angle while holding onto the back of the chair. Next, bring one foot in between the legs of the chair and then move into the pose. Repeat this sequence 10 times on one leg, holding the last Warrior 3 for a few seconds. Switch legs and repeat.

Bringing your foot towards the chair engages your abs. Warrior 3 itself improves balance, stability and enhances overall coordination. It targets muscles, including abs and lower back, work to maintain the straight line, building core strength. Warrior 3 also enhances focus and concentration, bringing mental clarity and mindfulness with regular practice.

6. STANDING TWIST 1

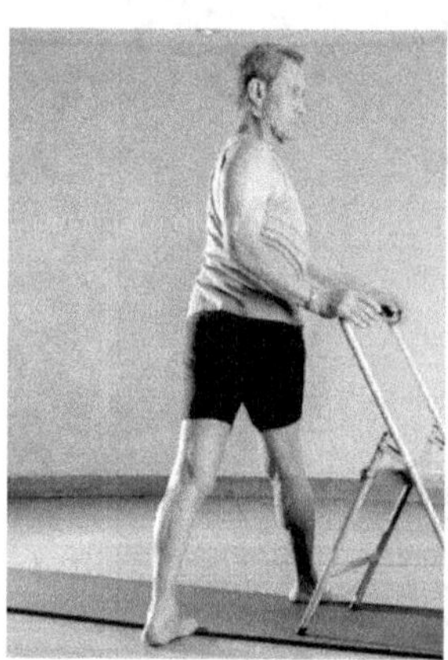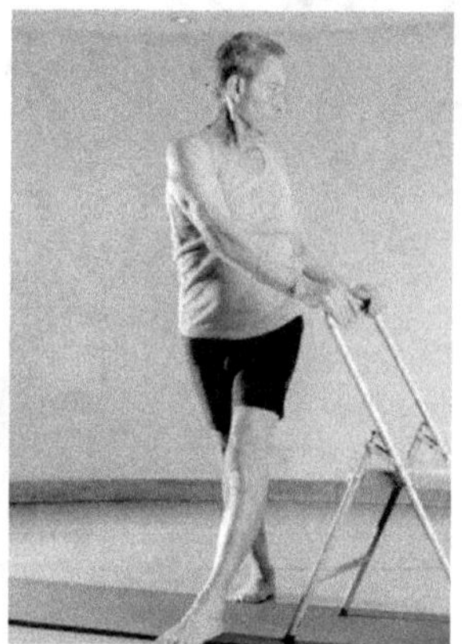

Even though this is a gentle twist -holding the back of the chair lightly and maintaining the pose for just a few seconds- it comes with many benefits. It´s great for spinal mobility, stretching the muscles and ligaments along the spine. Plus, it does wonders for digestive health by stimulating abdominal organs and aiding digestion. The twist also boosts balance, coordination, and proprioception. It promotes flexibility and mobility in the hips and shoulders.

Various muscles play a part in standing twists. The obliques on your torso´s sides, spinal erectors along the spine, and abdominals (rectus abdominis, transverse abdominis, and the obliques) stabilize the core during twists. The quadratus lumborum, located in the lower back helps with the twist, and the hip muscles also get in on the action.

7. SQUATS-1 (25 Reps minimum)

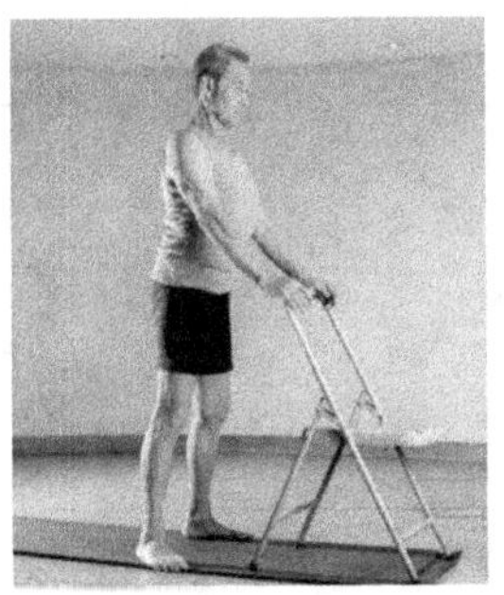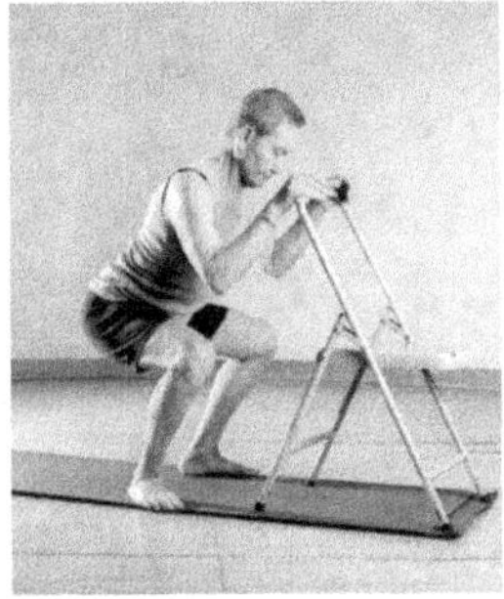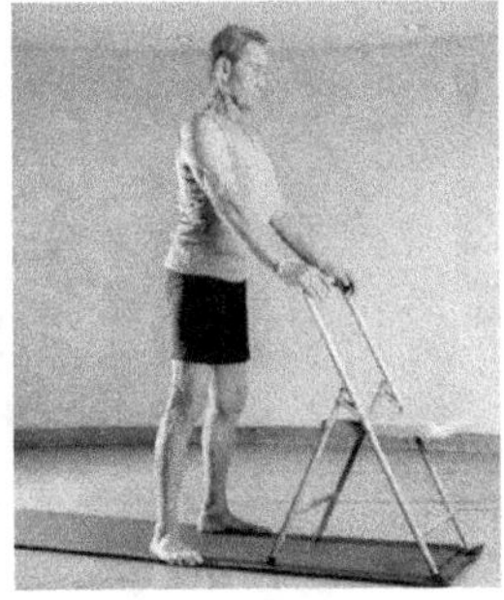

This exercise, a key part of the Yoga for Life routine, is done while holding onto the back of the chair and is repeated four times during the practice, with at least 25 reps each time. It´s not just a number – it´s because this move works wonders!

Here´s why: it strengthens leg muscles like quadriceps, hamstrings, adductors, and calves. Your core gets a workout engaging muscles in the abdomen and lower back. Plus, it builds gluteal muscles - the maximus, medius, and minimus. This squatting action is fantastic for overall fitness, burning calories promoting and promoting weight loss.

But, there´s more! This exercise boosts flexibility of your hip and ankle joints, and it´s a bone-density hero, crucial for your overall bone health. Let´s break down the muscles at play: quadriceps extend the knee, hamstrings flex it, gluteus muscles work hard, adductors on the inner thigh pitch in for hip adduction. The calves in the back of the lower leg are involved in ankle extension, calves extend ankle, and the core muscles keep the spine steady during the squat.

Now, about breathing – whether you inhale going down or exhale, it´s your call. Everyone´s different, but the key is to keep a steady and controlled rhythm throughout the exercise.

And, if possible, do the squats with eyes closed.

8. MOUNTAIN POSE-1 (10 Seconds)

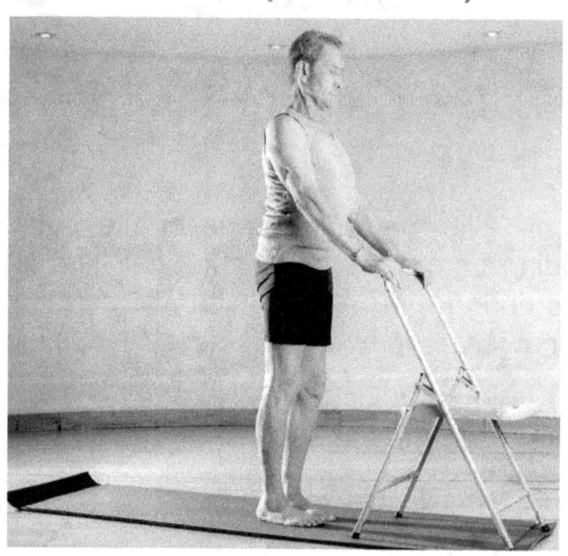

After finishing the squats, even though we hold the Mountain Pose for just ten seconds, pressing our heels against the ground while holding onto to the chair, "Tadasana" in Sanskrit, is a vital yoga pose that center and connect the mind and body. It is usually used as a starting or transitional pose in yoga sequences, and it sets the foundations for many standing and balancing poses. This pose puts emphasis on grounding, stability, and mindfulness. In Yoga for Life, we do it right after finishing squats to feel its effects and realign the whole body. Pressing the heels is key because it fully aligns your body.

Breathe evenly, keeping your focus on the breath to stay present in the moment. Holding the Mountain Pose improves overall posture, stability, and balance. Even though it may seem simple, it works various muscle groups, including the thighs, abdomen, and back muscles.

Remember to relax your shoulders, broaden your collarbones, and soften your gaze or close your eyes for a more soothing experience.

SECOND SECTION:
"CENTERING DOWN"

As we begin this section, the yawning and morning reluctance to work on yourself has already disappeared. Now is the perfect time to center your mind and let your consciousness expand through breathwork. Throughout ancient times, breath has been a trusted tool to sharpen the mind and guide us into thoughtful contemplation.

In some of the breathing exercises covered in this section, we highlight the importance of comfortably holding the breath on empty lungs for as long as possible. This practice is based on the understanding that this gas, carbon dioxide, plays a vital role in various physiological functions. It aids in regulating pH levels in the blood and contributes to the Bohr effect, facilitating the release of oxygen from hemoglobin in red blood cells.

Another objective in this second section is to stimulate the vagus nerve through diverse breathing patterns presented here. Additionally, the practice of mindfulness and relaxation can also have a positive impact on this important nerve.

Do not forget to press your tongue against the soft palate and slightly contract your pelvic floor.

9. DEEP SLOW BREATHS (30 Breaths minimum)

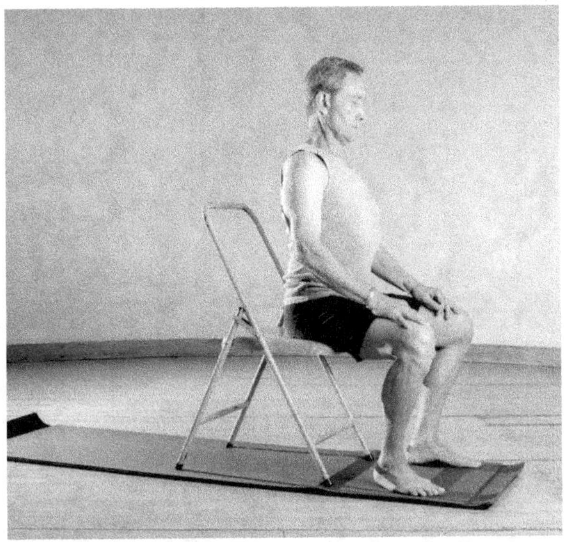

Sitting on the edge of the chair, feet firmly on the ground, spine straight, and hands resting on your thighs, keep your head aligned with the spine, and don´t forget to press your tongue against the soft palate.

If you´re familiar with yoga, you´ll gradually find yourself practicing "Ujjay breathing". Either way, engaging in deep, soft breathing brings mental and physiological benefits. Mentally, it promotes relaxation and reduces stress by calming the mind and fostering mindfulness. Physiologically, this type of breathing activates the parasympathetic nervous system, leading to a decrease in stress hormones like cortisol. This, in turn, lowers heart rate and blood pressure.

Moreover, deep breathing improves oxygen exchange in the lungs, supplying more oxygen to the body and brain, enhancing concentration and overall cognitive function. In a nutshell, practicing deep, soft breathing contributes to a feeling of calmness and balance in both mind and body.

10. SANKALPA-1

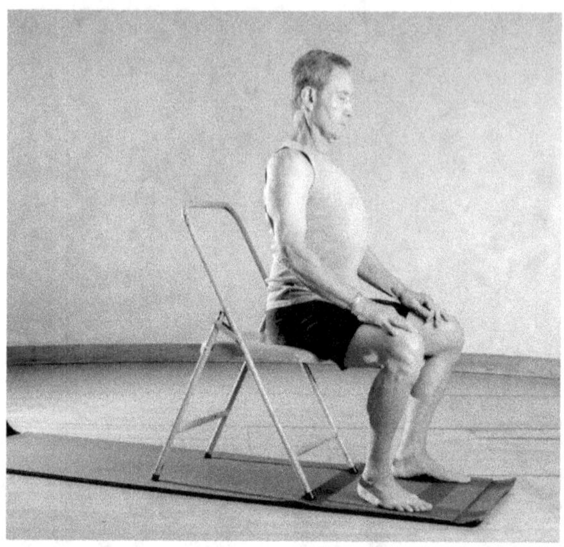

After a minute or so of gentle, deep breathing, your mind becomes calm. Now is the time for your ´Sankalpa´ - a sincere vow or commitment aligned with your true purpose and values. Mentally formulate it in present time, for example, "I´m healthy and happy", even if that is not your present reality. By regularly revisiting and reaffirming your ´Sankalpa´, this positive intention can bring about transformative changes in your life. Repeat your ´Sankalpa´ three times, keeping it short and clear.

11. KAPALABHATI: (54 Times)

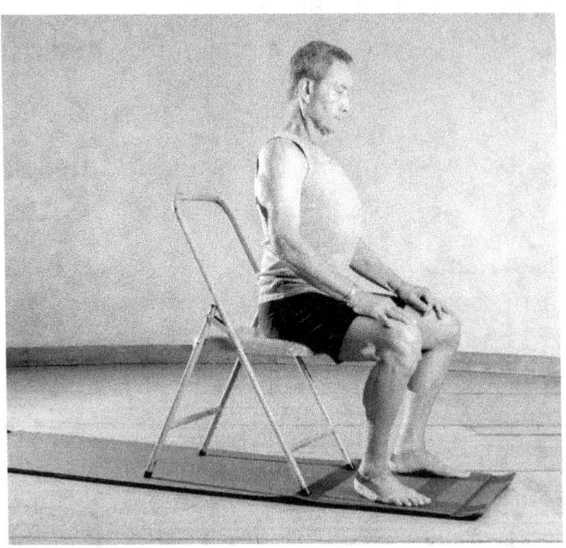

"Kapalabhati" is a breathing technique that involves rapid and forceful exhalations through the nose, while the inhalation occurs passively. The word ´Kapalabhati´ is often translated as ´shinning skull´ implying that one can achieve mental clarity through the practice of this Pranayama technique.

1. Sit comfortably with an upright spine and relaxed shoulders.

2. Take a deep breath in.

3. Exhale forcefully and quickly through the nose by contracting the abdominal muscles and the pelvic floor!

4. Allow inhalation to happen passively without any effort. Relax your pelvic floor!

5. Repeat this process in a rhythmic and rapid manner 54 times.

6. With the final exhale, hold your breath for as long as possible, tightening your pelvic floor muscles.

Subsequently, inhale and retain your breath for 10-15 seconds. Breathe normally and relax the tongue and pelvic floor while watching your mental screen.

Now, let´s explore some of the potential benefits of this technique:

The rapid exhalation of Kapalabhati help expel carbon dioxide from the lungs, allowing for a more efficient exchange of gases and increased oxygenation of the blood. The quick, forceful breaths stimulate the nervous system, promoting alertness and energizing the body. The forceful exhalations may help remove toxins from the lungs and body, supporting the detoxification process. Kapalabhati is believed to massage and stimulate the abdominal organs, promoting better digestion and elimination of waste. This type of breathing helps to clear the mind, and improve concentration. Also, strengthens the pelvic floor muscles.

12. BHASTRIKA 2 (54 Times)

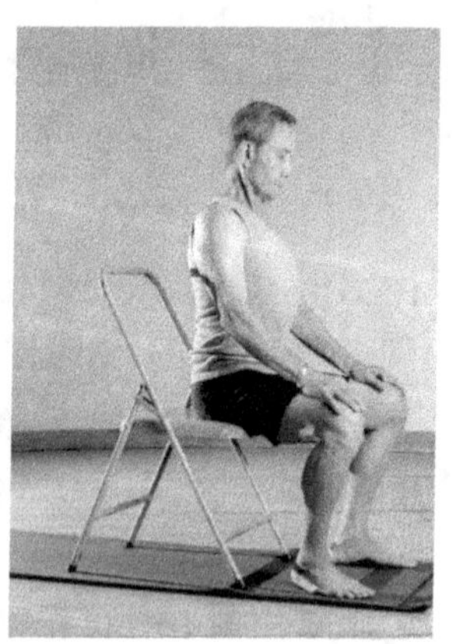 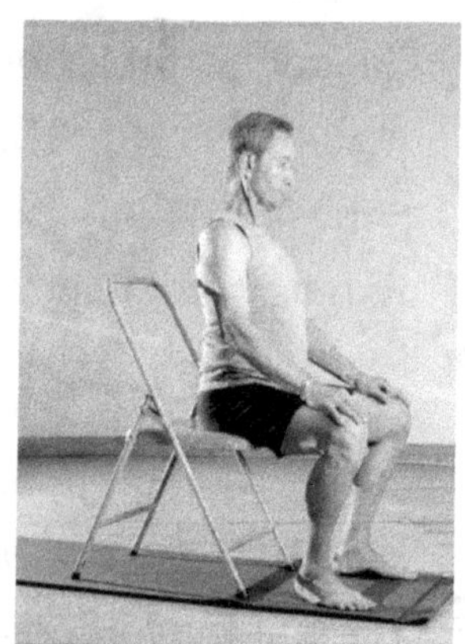

Often referred to as ´Bellows Breath´, is a dynamic and energizing yogic breathing technique. Rapid and forceful inhalations and exhalations are performed through the nose, creating a bellows-like effect. The breath is both vigorous and rhythmic, involving the expansion and contraction of the diaphragm.

Sit comfortably with an upright spine and relaxed shoulders. Take a deep breath in. Exhale by contracting the pelvic floor and abdominal muscles, and when inhaling, relax the pelvic floor and project your abdominal muscles outward. Repeat this process in a rhythmic and rapid manner 54 times. With the final exhale, hold your breath for as long as possible. Subsequently, inhale and retain your breath for 10-15 seconds. Breathe normally and relax the tongue and pelvic floor while watching your mental screen.

Though it may be challenging to discern, in the photo on the left, you will observe that my abdomen is near my spine, whereas in the photo on the right, my abdomen protrudes outwards.

Experience a range of benefits with this practice, including increased energy levels, improved respiratory function, cleansing and detoxification, stress reduction leading to enhanced well-being, heightened focus and mental clarity, increased strength in respiratory muscles for better overall respiratory health, and the strengthening of pelvic floor muscles to enhance core strength and support.

13. SQUATS-2 (25 Reps minimum)

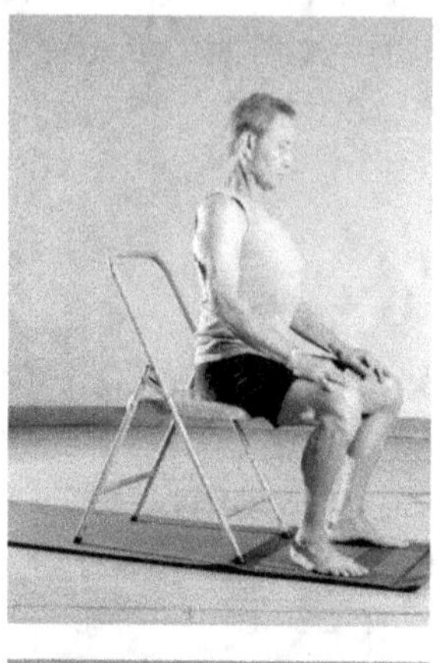
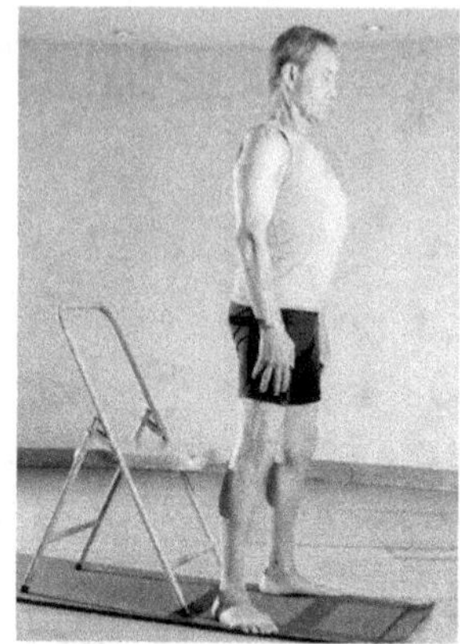
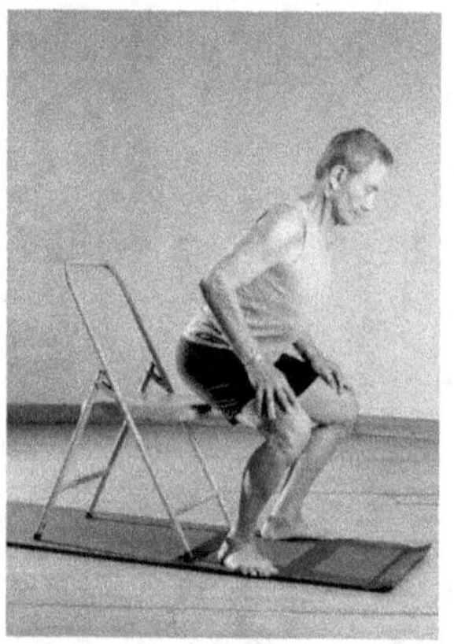
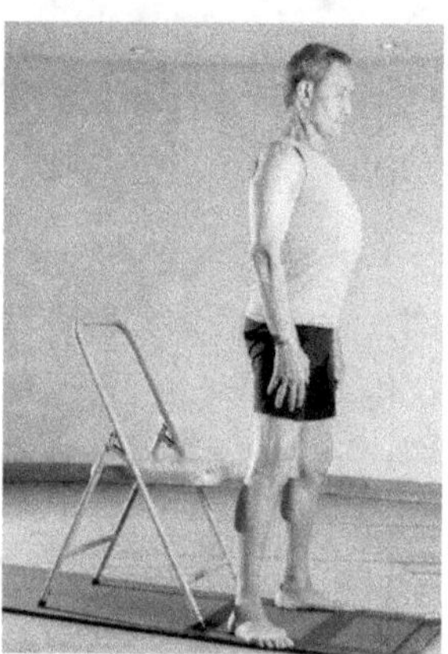

Here´s our second set of squats. This time, sit on the edge of the chair with the hands on your thighs. Let´s aim for at least 25 reps. We´ll incorporate two more squats in the same manner during this routine. The more squats we do, the stronger our legs become! And remember, if possible, do them with your eyes closed.

If you feel that doing squats in this manner does not suit you, do them as in the first section.

14. MOUNTAIN POSE-2 (10 Seconds)

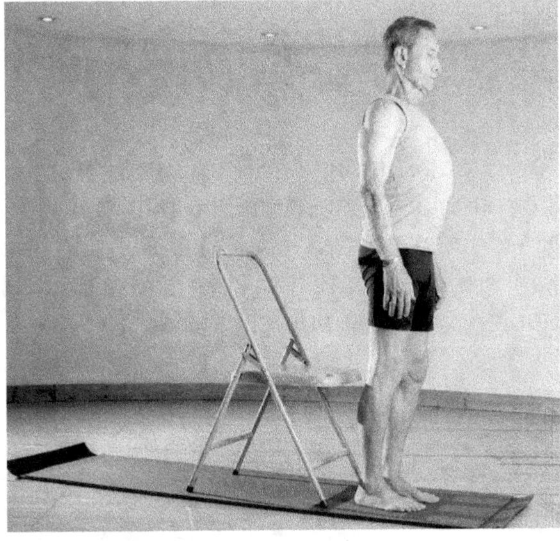

Similar to the previous Mountain Pose, this time we stand in front of the chair with our hands at the sides of the body, and the eyes closed.

THIRD SECTION:
"SOFT ACTIVATION OF THE SPINE"

Taking care of your spine is really important for your overall health. Your spine, also known as the backbone or vertebral column, is a crucial part of your skeleton. It does a lot of important things like supporting your body, letting you move around, and keeping your spinal cord safe - which is crucial for your nerves.

Here are some simple things to know about your spine:

1. **Number of Vertebrae:** Your spine is made up of 33 vertebrae.

2. **Cervical Spine (Neck):** The neck part of your spine is called the cervical spine, and it has seven vertebrae labeled C1 through C7. C1 is called the atlas, and C2 is called the axis. These vertebrae support the head, let you move your neck, and keep your spinal cord safe.

3. **Other Spine regions:** There are other parts of your spine too – the thoracic (upper and mid-back), lumbar (lower back), sacral (near the pelvis), and coccygeal (the tailbone).

4. **Intervertebral Discs:** Between the vertebrae, there are things called intervertebral discs. They work like shock absorbers, making sure the bones don´t rub against each other.

5. **Spinal Cord:** The spinal cord is super delicate and very important. It runs inside the vertebrae and helps messages travel between your brain and the rest of the body.

6. **Natural Curves:** Your spine has curves that help balance your body and spread it weight. There´s a

curve in your neck (cervical lordosis), one in your upper and mid-back (thoracic kyphosis), and one in your lower back (lumbar lordosis).

7. **Movement and Posture:** Your spine lets you move in lots of ways – you can bend, twist, and stand up straight because of it.

Remember, taking care of your spine is really important. In this section, we´ll start with some gentle exercises to keep it healthy and happy.

15. NECK 1, 2 & 3

It´s important to perform neck movements slowly and gently. A minute a day will keep your neck happy and healthy!

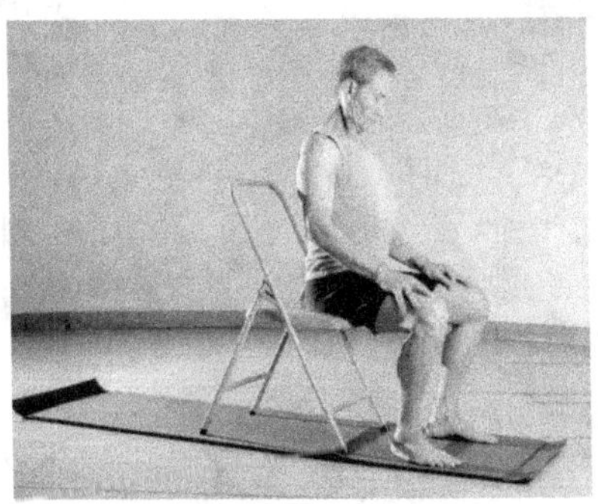
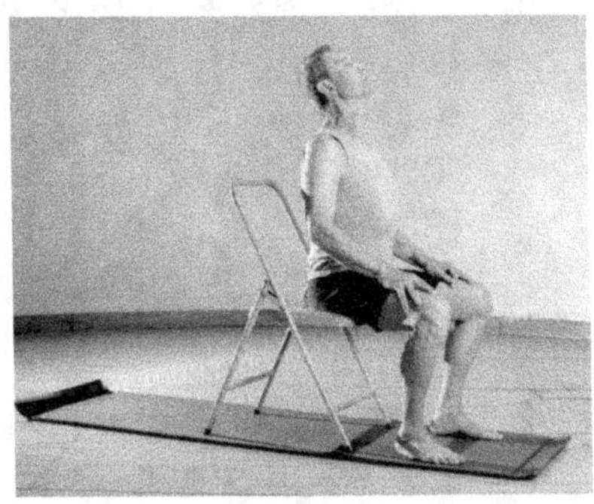

"Neck 1": Deep flexion and extension of the neck.

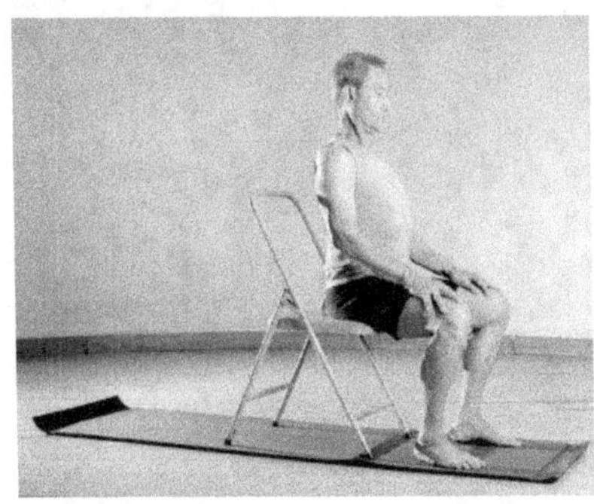
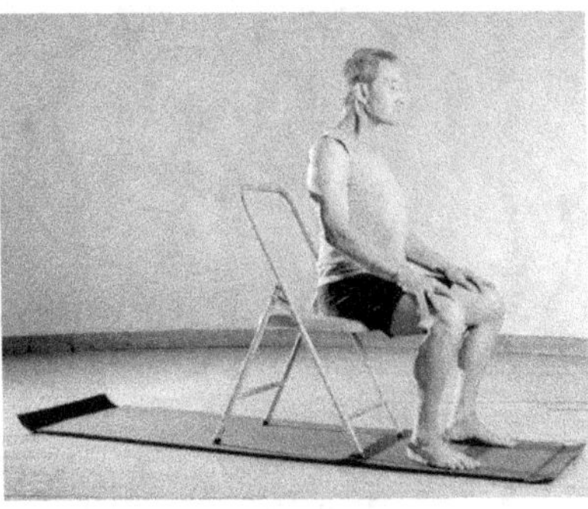

"Neck 2": Moving the neck back and forth.

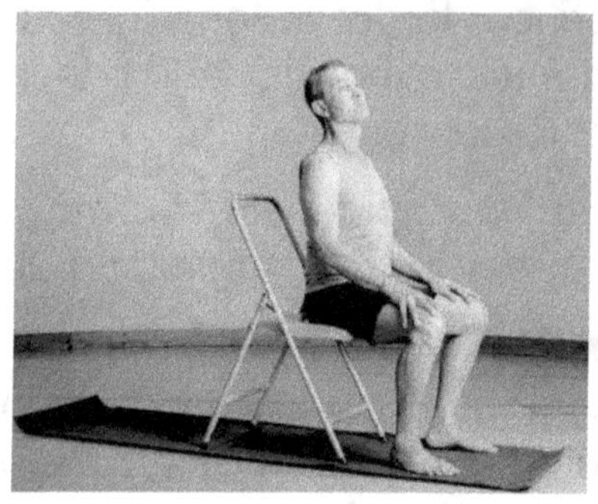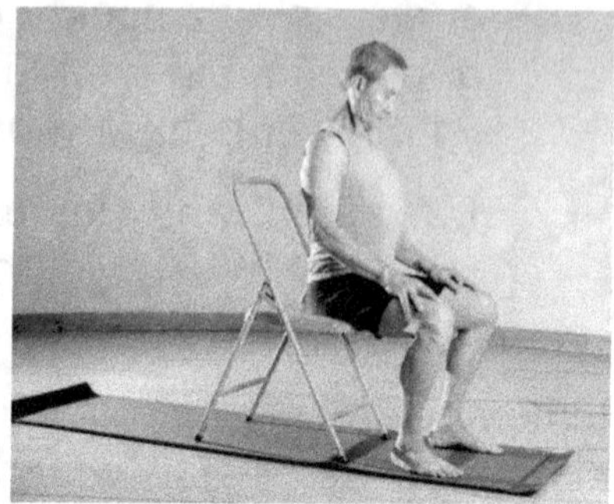

"**Neck 3**": Neck rotations.

These three easy neck exercises are done in less than a minute and are very beneficial for several reasons:

1. **Vagus Nerve Stimulation:** This nerve also known as the tenth cranial nerve, plays a crucial role in the parasympathetic nervous system, which is responsible for the "rest and digest" response. Stimulation of the vagus nerve has been associated with various health benefits, including relaxation, stress reduction, and improved overall well-being.

2. **Increased Flexibility:** Regular neck movements help improve flexibility of the neck muscles and joints and reduce stiffness.

3. **Release of Tension:** Neck movements help release tension in the neck and upper shoulder area.

4. **Improved Circulation:** These exercises can enhance blood circulation to the neck muscles and surrounding tissues.

5. **Prevention of Stiffness:** Poor posture or sleeping in an uncomfortable position can contribute to neck stiffness.

6. **Enhanced Posture Awareness:** Performing neck exercises encourages awareness of proper neck and

head alignment. This awareness can translate into improved posture in daily activities.

7. **Strengthening Muscles:** Controlled neck movements can contribute to the strengthening of neck muscles providing better support to the head and neck.

16. SIDEWAYS LEANING

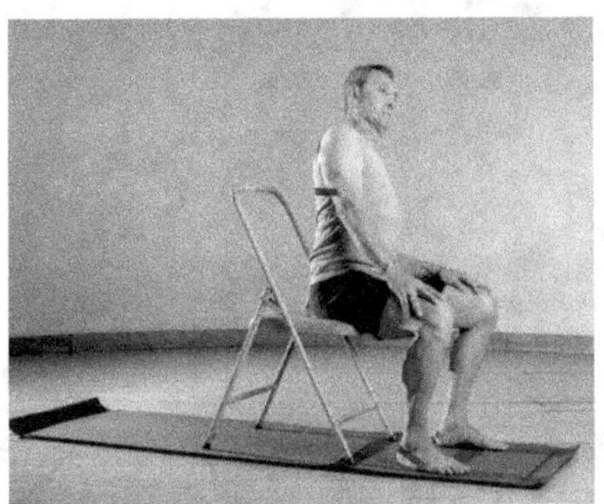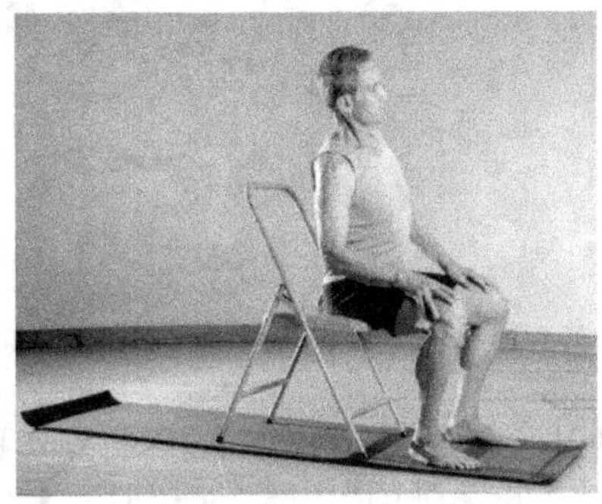

For this exercise, keep sitting on the edge of the chair and gently lean your body first to one side, then to the other, while keeping your head in line with your spine. Be sure not to lift the opposite buttock. Exhale as you lean to the sides, and inhale as your return to the center.

This soothing exercise offers a delightful stretch for your spine and engages various muscles. The muscles involved in this action includes those along your sides, known as the obliques, which help with lateral movements and core stability. By incorporating sideways leaning into your routine, you promote flexibility, release tension, and support a healthy posture.

Repeat this exercise two or three times on each side.

17. LIGHT TWIST-2

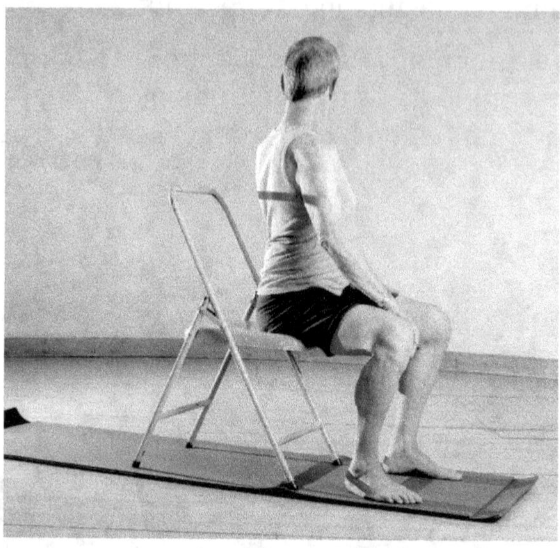

This second twist is gentler and more soothing than the one we did in the first section. The benefits are similar. Repeat two or three times on each side.

18. LOOKING FOR A FLY

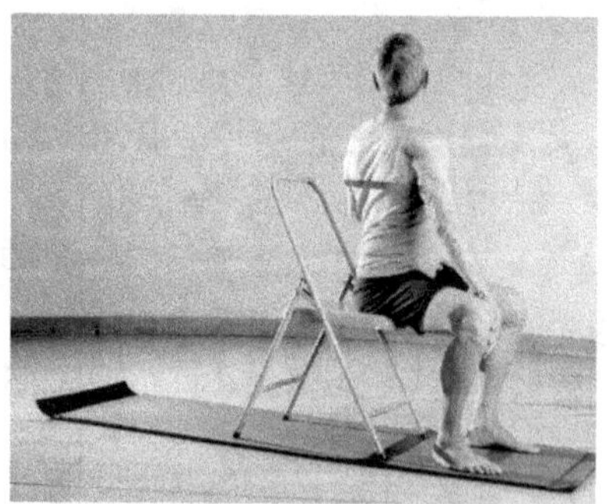 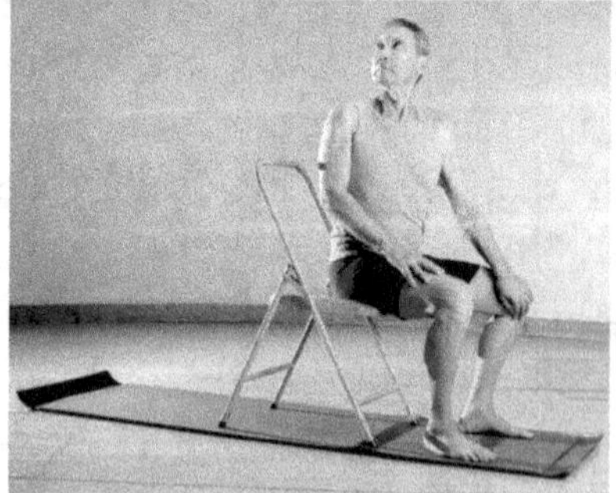

This is also a gently twist. The only difference with the previous one, is that we look over the shoulder towards the ceiling, like looking for a fly. The benefits of all the twists are similar. Repeat this exercise two times.

19. PELVIC ANTEVERSION AND RETROVERSION

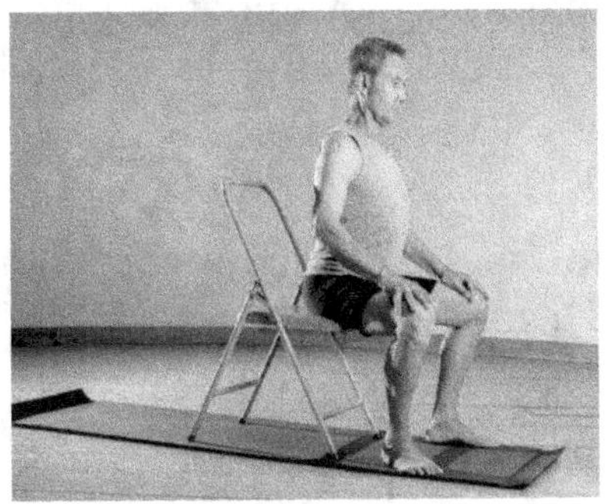 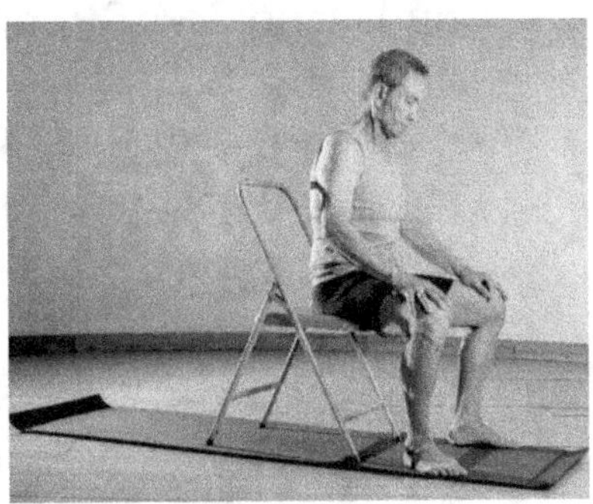

Anteversion and retroversion refers to how the pelvis tilts in relation to the rest of the body. Both are normal movements that can vary among individuals, affecting posture, comfort, movements patterns, and potential musculoskeletal issues. Tilted pelvis is a technique used in GPBALANCE for its great benefits.

Pelvic Anteversion: Occurs when the pelvis is tilted forward. In simpler terms, the front part of the pelvis moves downwards, and the back part moves upwards. It is the typical position of the pelvis when standing or walking.

Pelvic Retroversion: Is the opposite of anteversion. It occurs when the pelvis is tilted backwards. In this case, the back part of the pelvis moves downward, and the front part moves upwards. It is associated with a flattened lower back.

Tilting the pelvis back and forth, or incorporating movements that involve pelvic anteversion and retroversion, can offer various benefits, especially when done mindfully and as a part of a well-rounded approach to movement and exercise. Here are some potential benefits:

1. **Improved Posture:** Awareness of pelvic positioning is essential for maintaining a neutral spine and reducing the risk of postural issues.

2. **Enhanced Core Strength:** Pelvic movements engage the muscles of the core, including the abdominal muscles and lower back.

3. **Flexibility and Mobility:** Tilting the pelvis back and forth promotes flexibility and mobility in the hip joints and lower back. This is particularly beneficial for people who experience stiffness in these areas.

4. **Prevention of Lower Back Pain:** Contribute to a more balanced distribution of forces across the spine and pelvis.

5. **Muscle Activation:** Tilting the pelvis activates various muscles, including the hip flexors, hamstrings, and glutes. This activation contributes to muscle balance and may reduce the risk of muscle imbalances that can lead to discomfort or injury.

6. **Improved Circulation:** Dynamic pelvic movement can enhance blood circulation in the pelvic region and lower back, providing nutrients to the muscles and supporting overall tissue health.

7. **Core Awareness:** The awareness we acquire doing this exercise translate into improved body mechanics during daily activities.

8. **Relaxation and Stress Reduction:** Mindful movements, especially when coordinated with the breath, can have a calming effect on the nervous system.

Do this exercise at least 20 to 30 times. On the retroversion, contract your pelvic floor muscles and on the anteversion, relax them. Keep the tongue pressing the soft palate during the exercise.

20. EXPANSION AND CONTRACTION OF THE SPINE

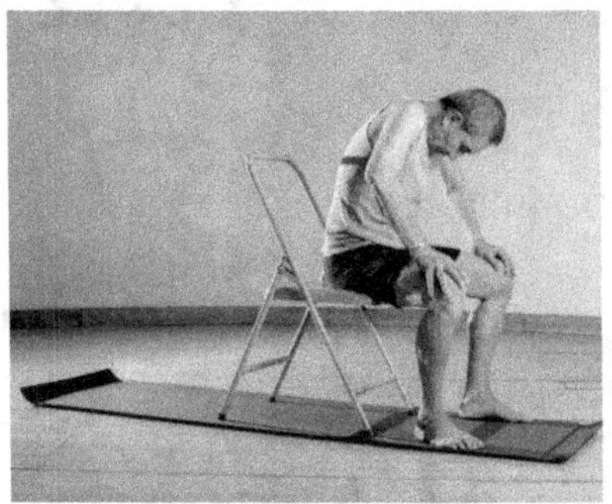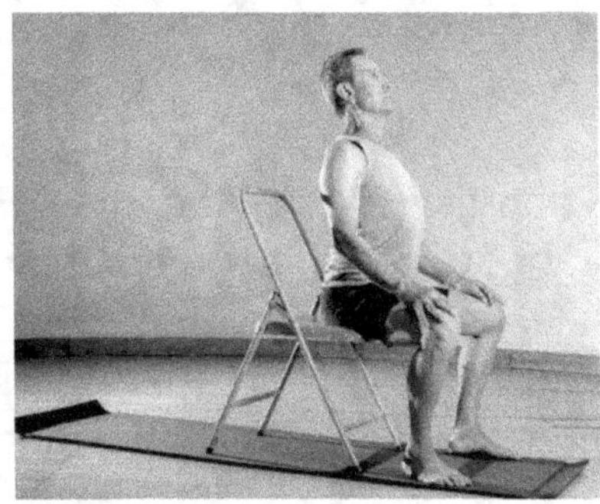

Sit on the edge of the chair with your back straight. Exhale as you gently lower your head towards your knees, feeling your back rounding and your spine stretching. Inhale and return opening your chest and tilting your head slightly backward. Repeat this movement at least three times. Potential benefits may include improved posture, reduced tension, and enhanced flexibility of the spine.

This is one of the initial movements for the spine we do in yoga; albeit performed in a different position, than the typical hands and knees on the ground. These postures are commonly called as the "cat" and "cow" positions.

21. FULL ROTATION OF THE TRUNK

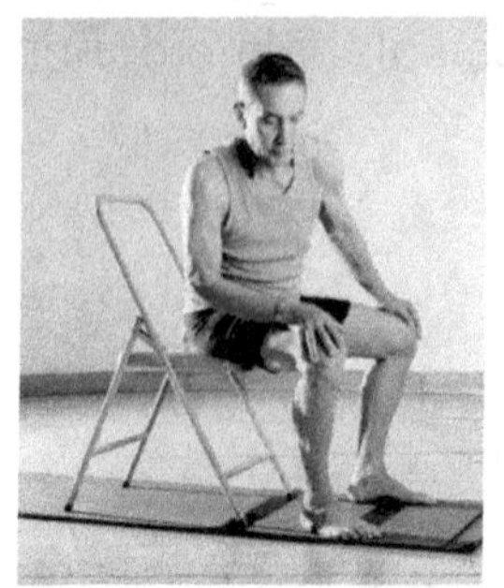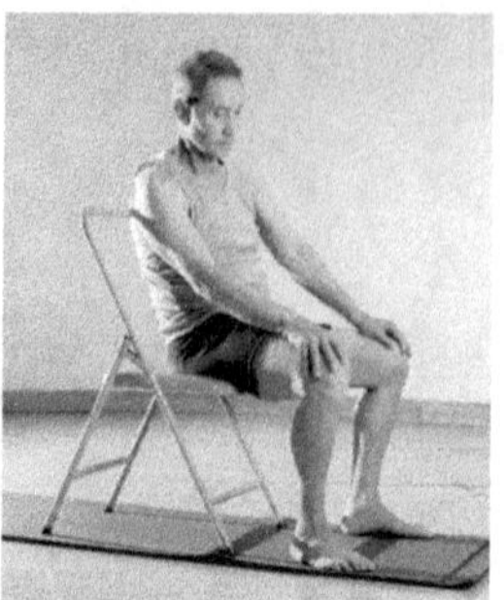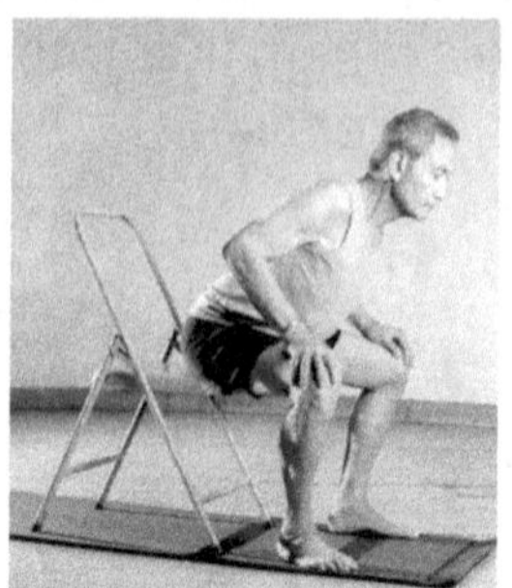

Sit on the edge of the chair. Rotating your trunk brings lots of body benefits: better spine movement, stronger core, balanced muscles, improved posture, more flexibility, relief from tension, and mind-body connection. Do this move three times on each side, matching it with the breath.

22. SQUATS-3 (25 Reps minimum)

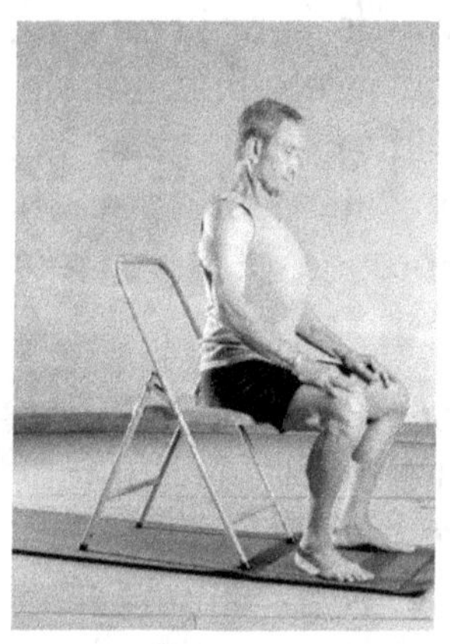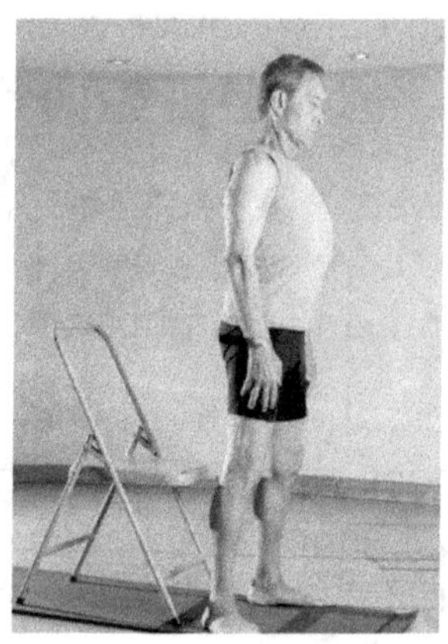

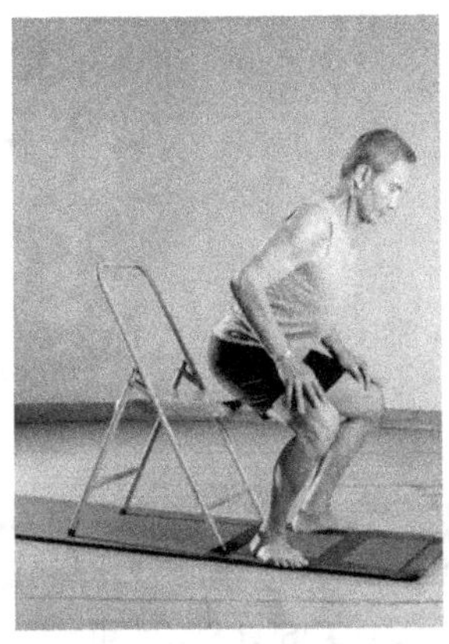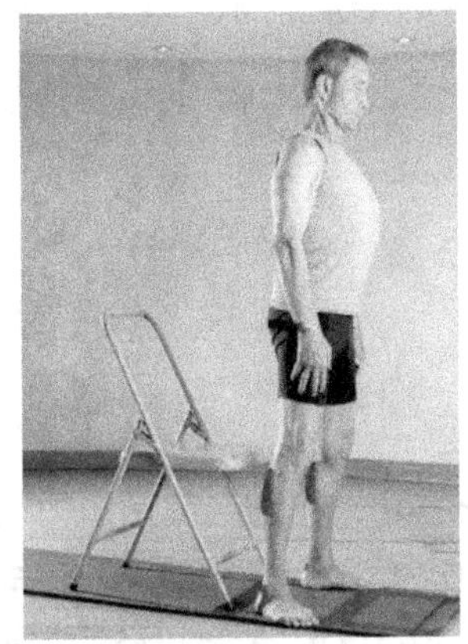

Here´s our third set of squats. Let´s aim for at least 25 reps. We´ll do just one more squat in the same way during this routine. The more squats we do, the stronger our legs become! And remember, if possible, do them with eyes closed.

23. MOUNTAIN POSE-3 (10 Seconds)

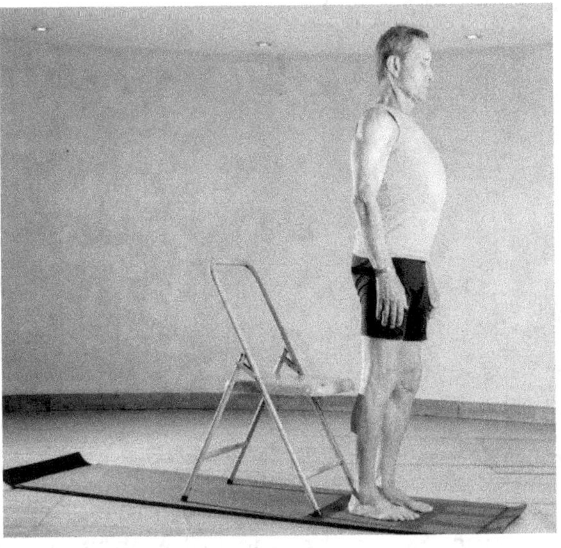

Same as the one we did on the second section. If possible, keep your eyes closed.

FOURTH SECTION: "FULL ACTIVATION OF THE SPINE AND MAIN JOINTS".

In the preceding section, we emphasized the significance of engaging in comprehensive spine movements. Failing to move or neglecting exercises that target this central axis can leave our bodies vulnerable to various discomforts and potential health issues. These may include deformities like scoliosis, kyphosis, and lordosis, which involve abnormal curvatures of the spine. Additionally, issues such as disc herniation, degenerative diseases, and spinal stenosis are common problems associated with intervertebral discs. Neglecting spine health may also contribute to the collapse of the spine and shortening. Regular, intentional movement and exercises targeting the spine are crucial for maintaining its health and preventing these potential complications.

24. DYNAMIC TWIST-3

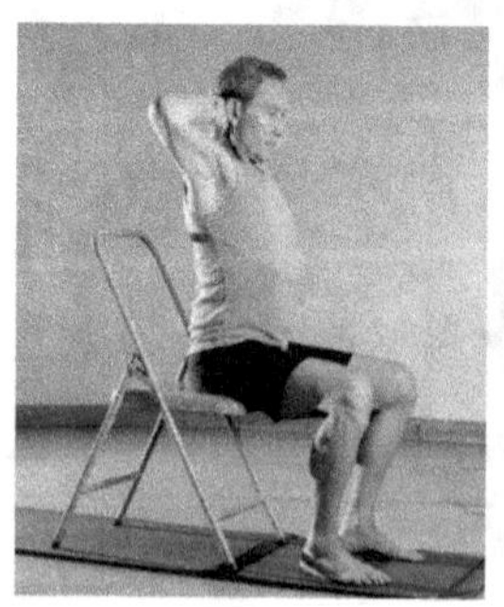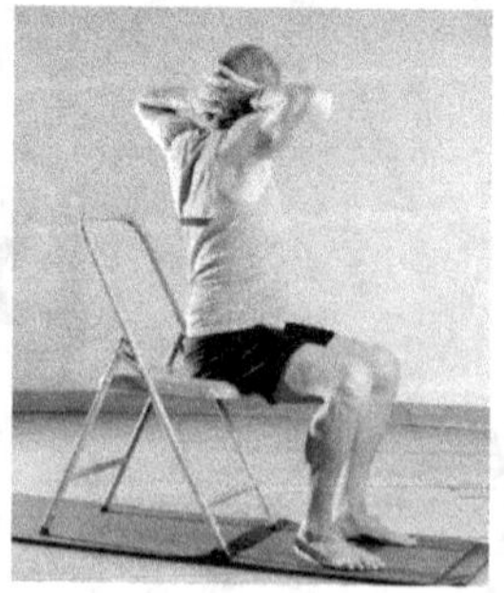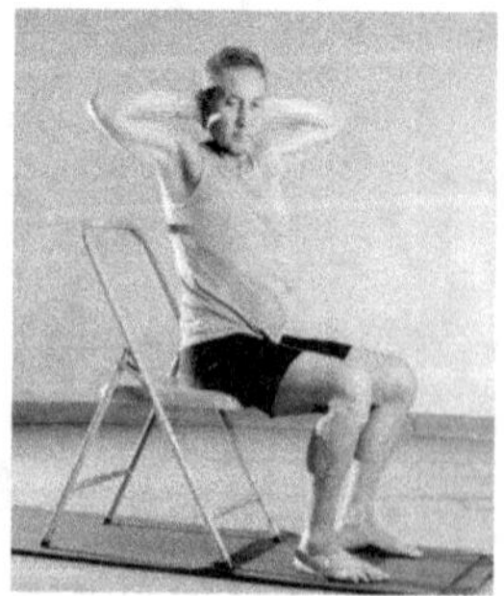

Give this quick twist a try for a boost in your day! Here's a simple technique: Sit on the edge of a chair, interlock your hands behind your head, and open your elbows. Inhale as you turn one way, exhale as you turn the other—repeat at least 27 times. Keep your tongue on the soft palate and gently contract the pelvic floor. Afterward, stretch your interlocked hands toward the ceiling with palms facing up.

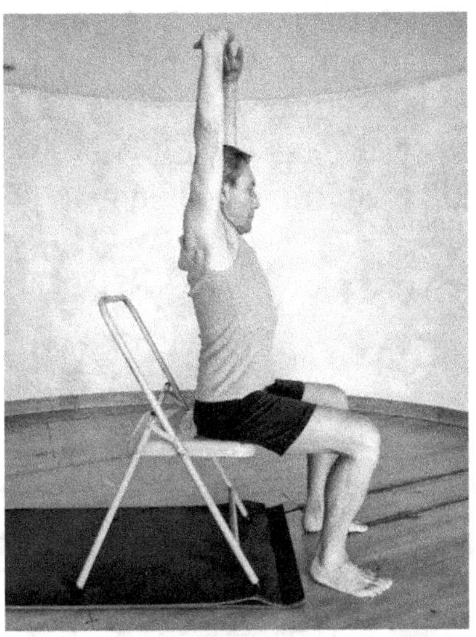

This practice comes with several perks, including increased flexibility, improved posture, and a refreshing energy boost!

25. ELBOW TO HIP

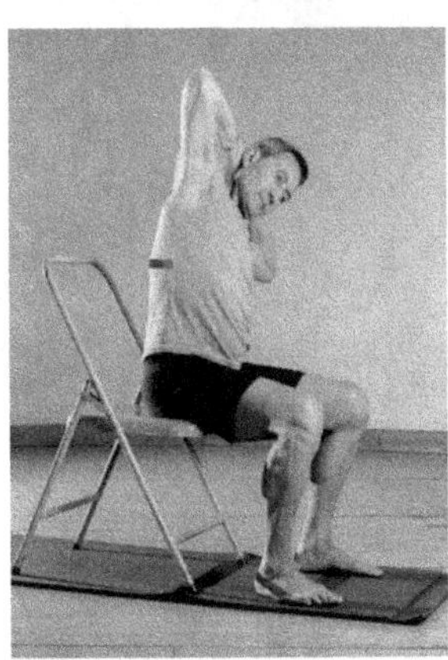

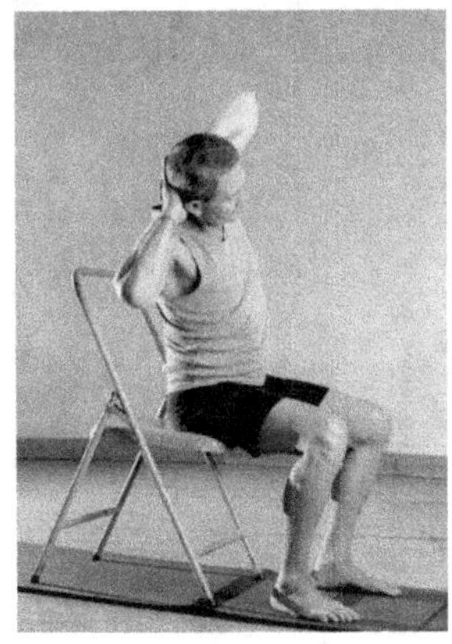

Clasp your hands behind your head, as in the previous technique, while sitting on the edge of the chair. Ensure your elbows are wide open. Inhale, and as you exhale, bring one elbow towards the hip; inhale as you return. Repeat on the other side. Maintain a rhythmic flow by repeating this movement several times. Keep your tongue on the soft palate and slightly contract the pelvic floor. Afterward, stretch your interlocked hands toward the ceiling with palms facing up.

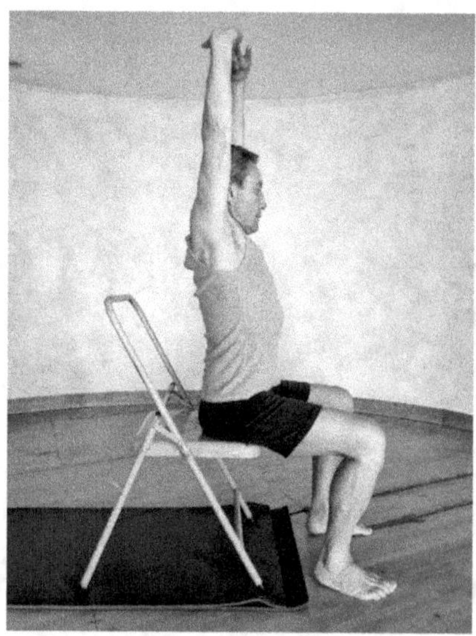

This exercise improves your spine flexibility, enhances posture, and strengthens core.

26. ELBOW TO KNEE

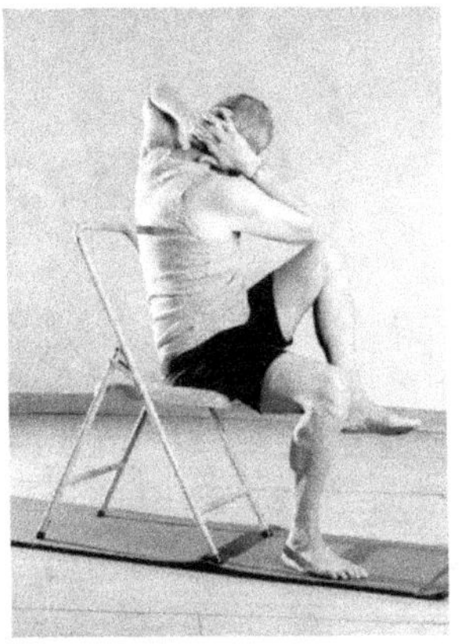 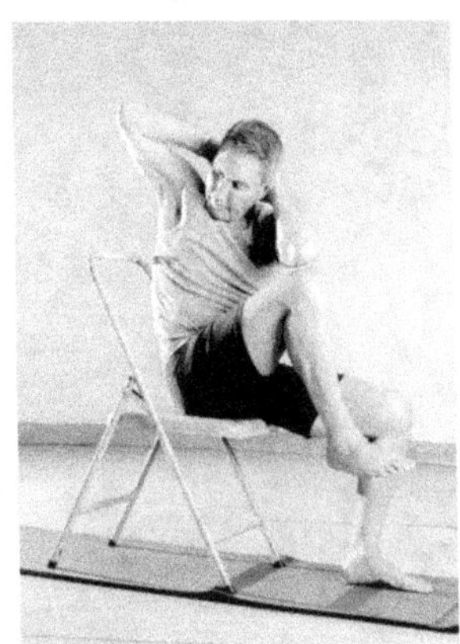

This technique involves a twist and a contraction of the abdominal muscles, making it excellent for revitalizing the spine, internal organs, and core. The more times you perform it, the better! After completing the exercise, stretch your interlocked hands toward the ceiling with palms facing up.

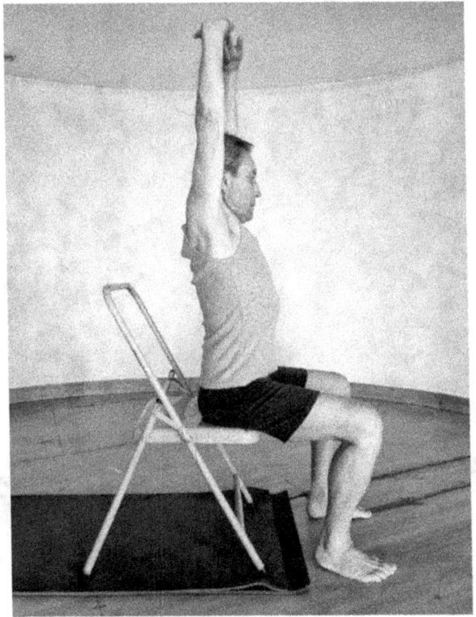

27. HAND TO FOOT

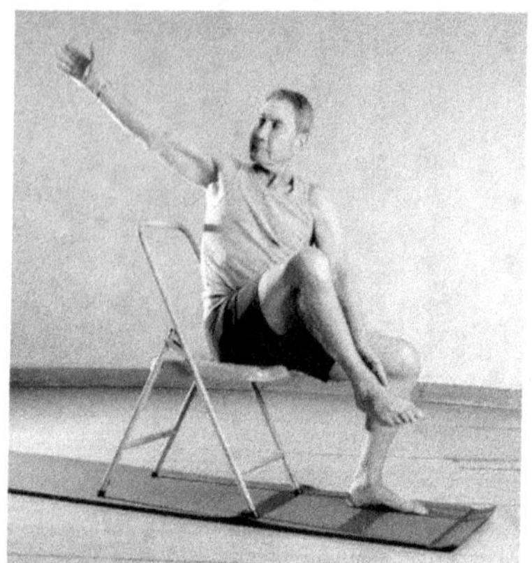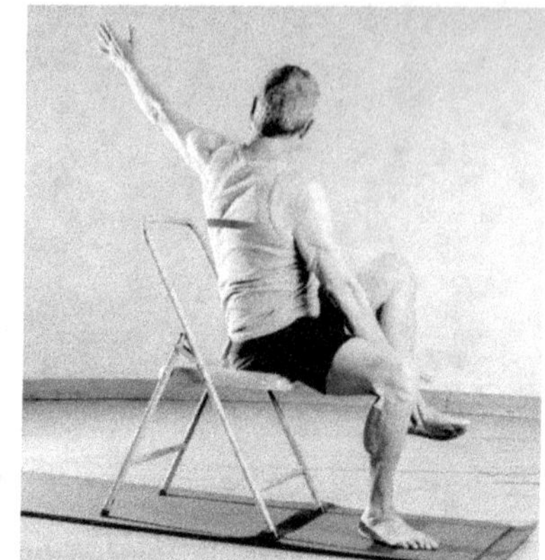

Sit on the edge of the chair. Bring one hand to the opposite foot while lifting the opposite arm backward. This exercise not only twist your spine, but also works your upper body and shoulder muscles, engaging the oblique muscles in your core.

28. SQUATS-4 (25 Reps minimum)

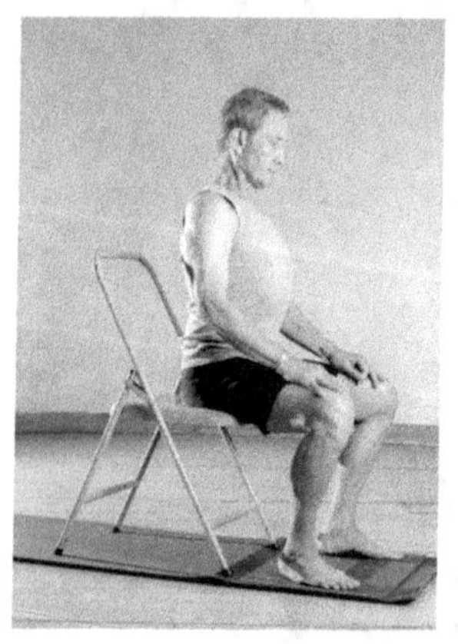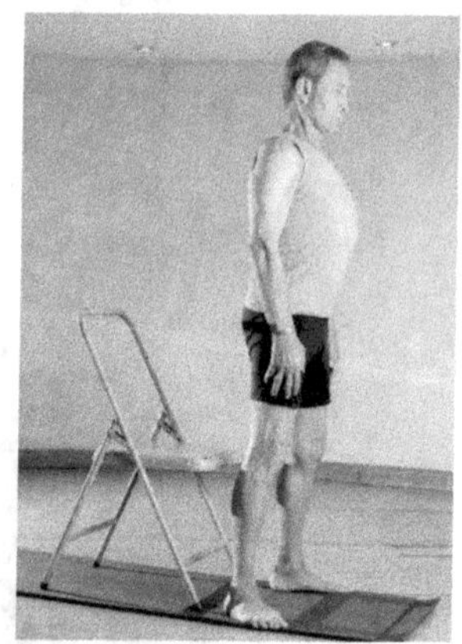

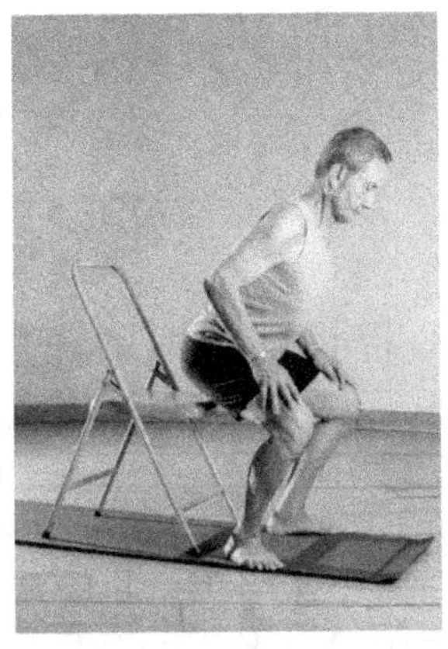 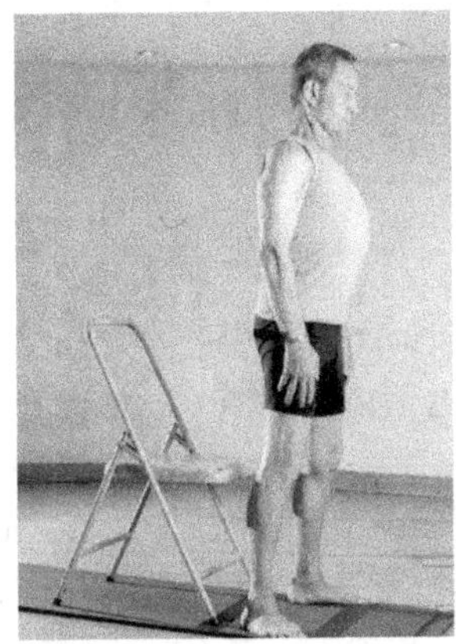

Here´s our four and last set of squats. Let´s aim for at least 25 reps. Remember: the more squats we do, the stronger our legs become!

29. MOUNTAIN POSE-4 (10 Seconds)

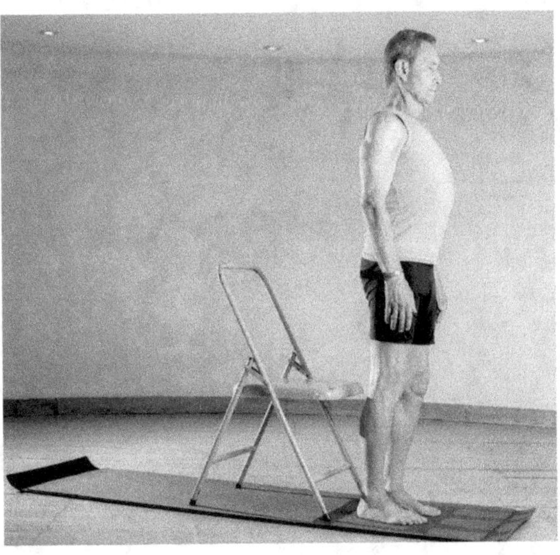

This is our last Mountain Pose. If possible, keep your eyes closed.

FIFTH SECTION: "STRENTHENING LEGS, ARMS, BACK AND ABDOMEN"

This part of the routine can be challenging because it works the whole body, especially the core, legs, arms and back, making you break a sweat. The number of repetitions is intentionally kept moderate, giving you the flexibility to increase them as you become stronger. The standing poses in this section are common in Hatha Yoga. To maximize their benefits, aim to hold each pose a little longer.

30. ABDOMINALS-1 (25 Reps with each leg)

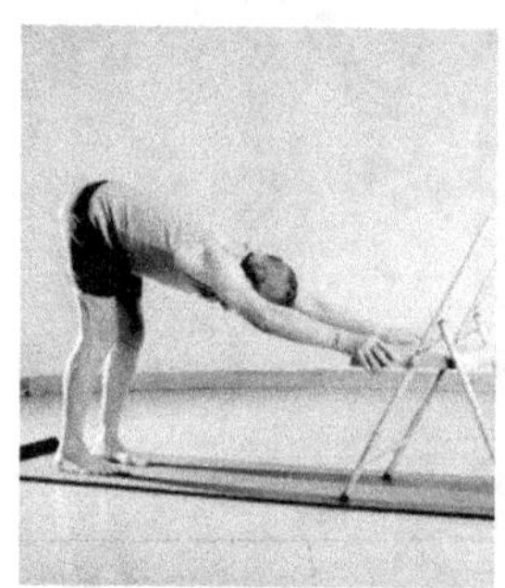
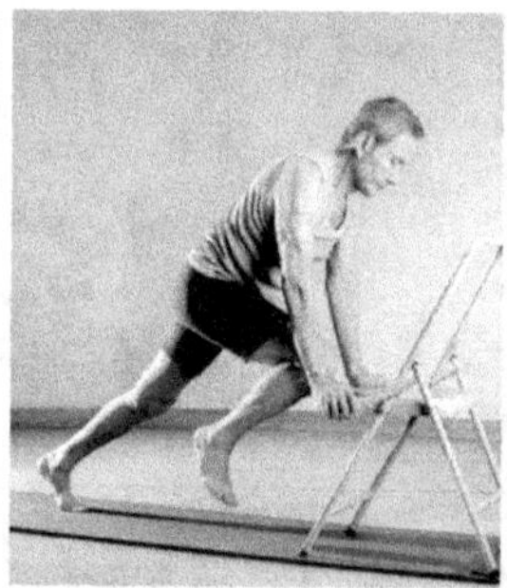
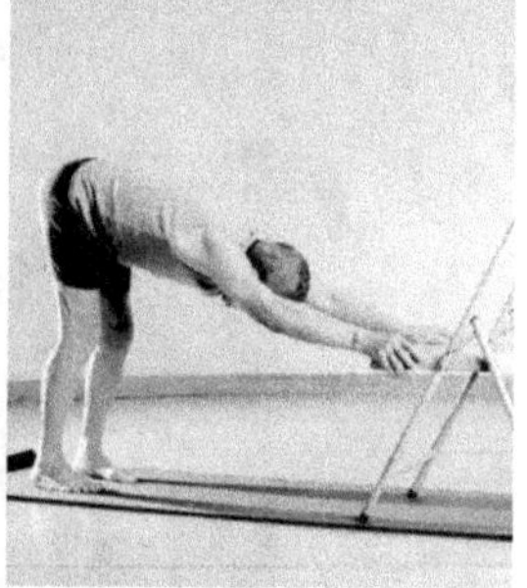

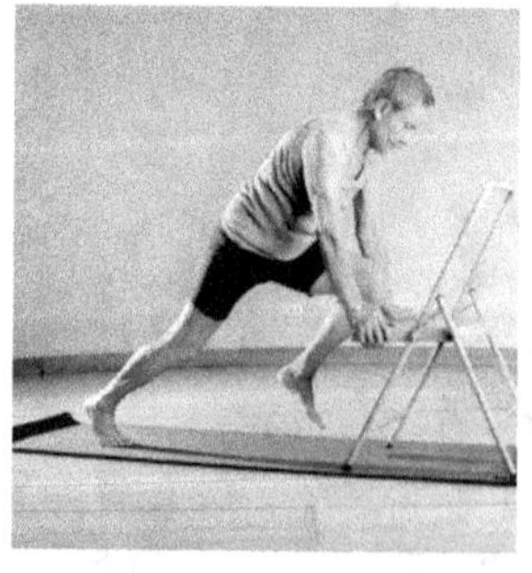
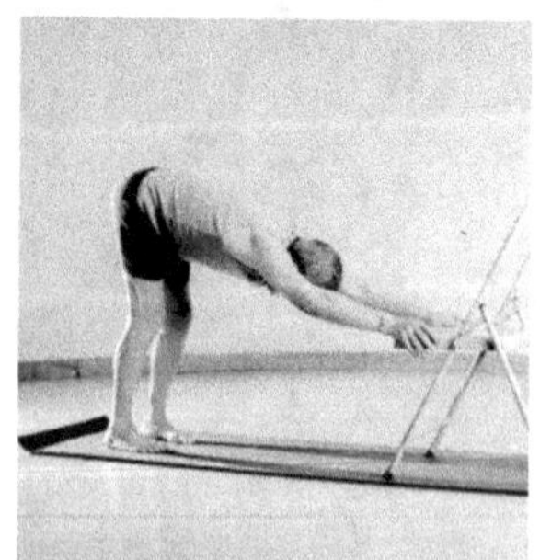

This exercise is highly effective for targeting your abdominal muscles! Additionally, it provides a good stretch for your spine and the back of your legs. Whether you prefer a slow, controlled pace, a more deliberate approach, or a faster workout when time is limited, this routine can be tailored to your needs.

To perform the exercise, start by stretching your body as shown in the first picture. Bring your right knee toward the chair, then return to the starting position while stretching your body. Repeat the same movement with your left leg, ensuring you don´t touch the floor.

For optimal results, consider increasing the repetitions gradually as your core strength improves.

31. HIGH LUNGE-UTTHITA TRIKONASANA-VIRABHADRASANA II (1ST SIDE)

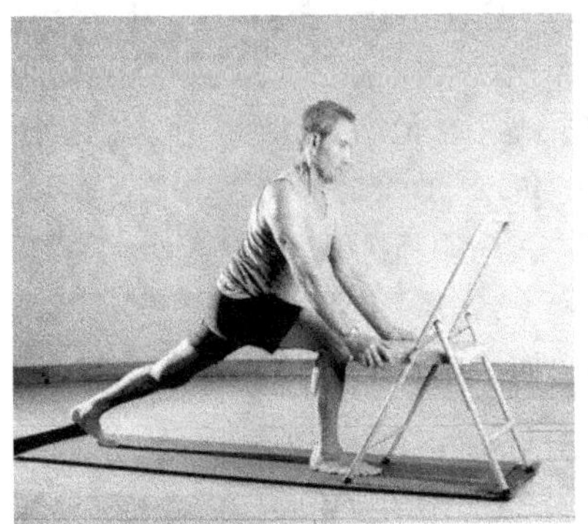

High Lunge

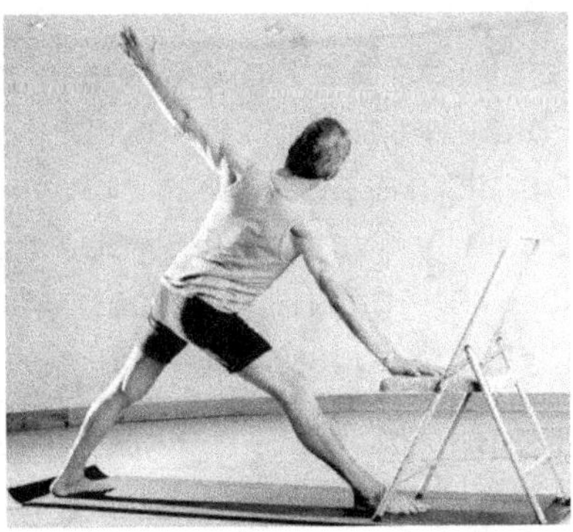

Utthita Trikonasana

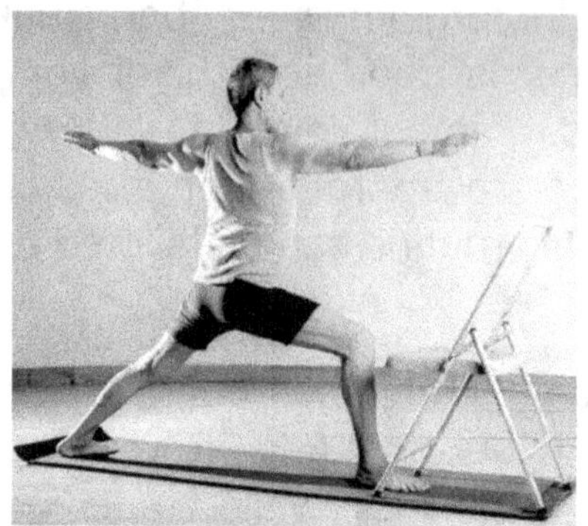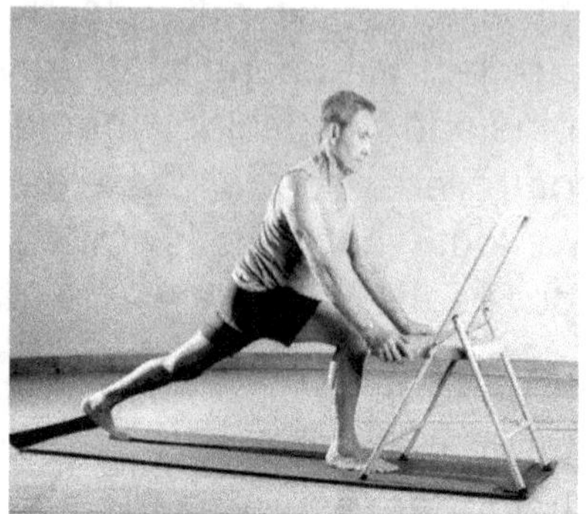

Virabhadrasana II

Try these three techniques one after the other. Each has its own benefits. If you can, stay in each one as long as you can – that´s the secret to getting the most out of each pose. Let's start with the first one: High Lunge.

High Lunge is great for your body and mind. It makes your legs muscles, like the quadriceps, hamstrings, and calf muscles stronger. It also works your core, making you more stable. This pose gives a good stretch to your hip flexors, which is especially helpful if you sit a lot or have tight hips. It´s also a pose that can give you more energy. Doing it regularly can make your hips, thighs, and ankles more flexible. And the best part: it gets your body ready for more advanced poses, like the next one: Utthita Trikonasana.

Utthita Trikonasana, also known as Extended Triangle Pose, offers various physical and mental benefits. Promotes more flexibility and strength in the lower body. As this pose involves a wide stance, it helps to open and stretch the hips and groin area, which can be especially beneficial for individuals with tightness in these areas. This pose involves a lateral stretch, enhancing flexibility in the spine promoting better posture. The twist in the torse stimulates the abdominal organs, aiding digestions and promoting overall abdominal health. This pose challenges your balance, improving coordination and stability. Utthita Trikonasana can provide relief from a mild backache because it relieves tension in the lower back. The stretching and twisting motions in this pose can help stimulate blood circulation throughout the body, bring fresh oxygen to various organs and tissues. The combination of mindful breathing and the physical aspects of the pose can help reduce stress and anxiety. Also, improves concentration.

Let´s explore now **Virabhadrasana II**, also known as Warrior II - a foundational yoga pose that brings a variety of benefits for your body and mind. This pose is excellent for strengthening your legs muscles –quadriceps, hamstrings, and calves– while toning and defining them. With its wide stance, Warrior II opens up your hips, providing relief especially if you spend a lot of time sitting. Regular practice can enhance balance and stability.

Beyond physical strength, regular practice of Warrior II contributes to improved balance and stability. Holding the pose for an extended period enhances endurance and stamina. This yoga pose encourages a focused mind aiding mental clarity and mindfulness.

The expansive posture of Warrior II, with an open chest and extended arms, promotes deep breathing expanding respiratory function, and increasing lung capacity. Additionally, it fosters good posture, helping you stand tall and straight.

32. PUSH UPS-1 (10-25 Reps) – URHVAMUKHA-ADHOMUKHA (10 Reps)

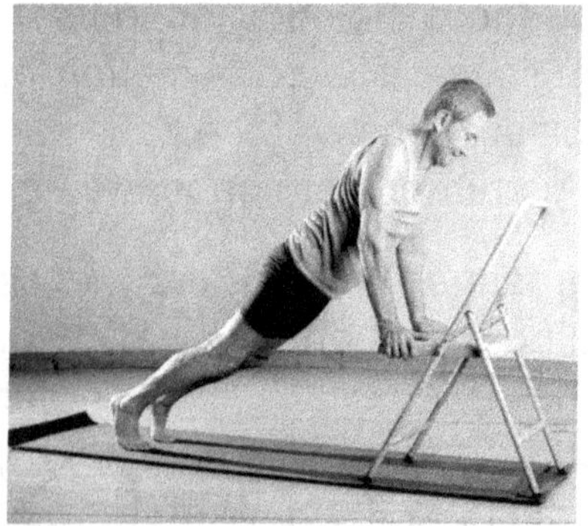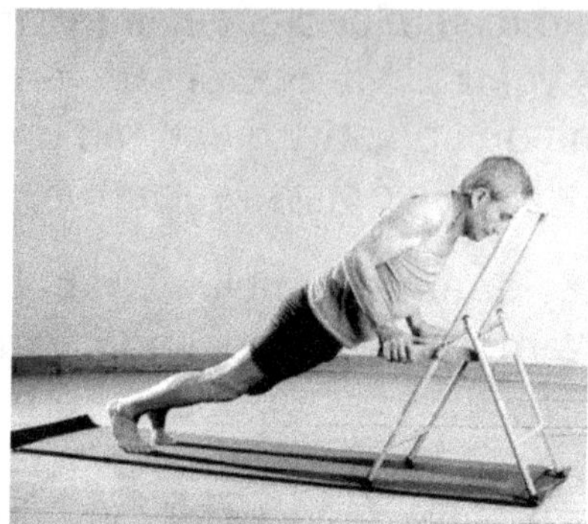

Push-ups

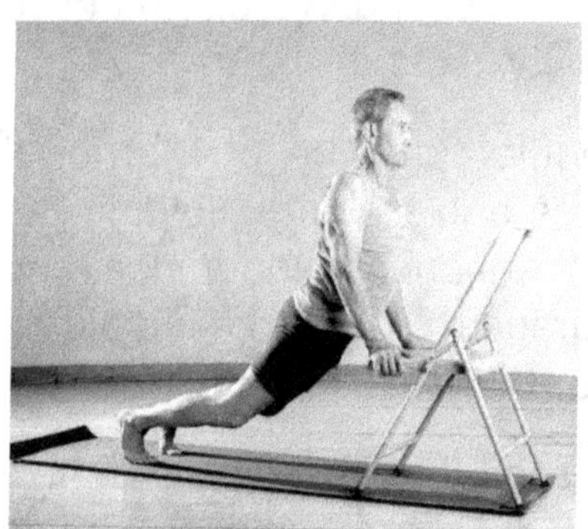

Urdhva Mukha

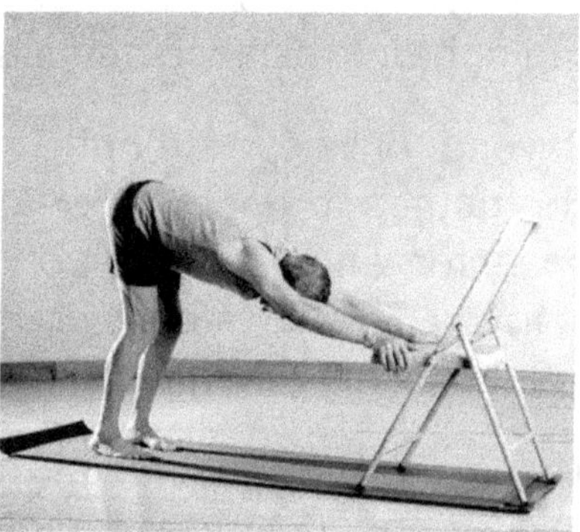

Adho Mukha

Push-ups are pretty straightforward and popular because they bring overall strength, endurance and boost functional fitness. Now, in my approach, we do them with a little twist - hands on a chair. It´s simpler, making it more likely you you´ll give it a go!

Let´s dive into why push-ups are so cool:

Push-ups mainly target your upper body muscles like the chest, shoulders, and triceps. They also engage you core muscles, making you more stable and stronger. Regular push-ups can enhance your endurance and contribute to stable shoulder blades, promoting better shoulder health. Plus, they're good for your wrists, elbows, and overall joint wellbeing.

The muscles doing the heavy lifting during push-ups include the chest muscles, shoulder muscles, and triceps. And don´t forget about the back muscles like the rhomboids and trapezius – they get a workout too!

After doing pushups (the more the better), we move on to the usual Urdhva Mukha-Adho Mukha sequence - 10 times. In Yoga for Life I have adjusted them to be done with a chair. Now, let´s explore the benefits of Urdhva Muka Svanasana first.

Urdhva Mukha Svanasana, or Upward-Facing Dog Pose, offers many benefits and engage multiple muscles groups. It strengthens the spine by lifting and opening the chest. This pose also stretches the lungs, promoting better breathing, and stimulates the abdominal organs. Urdhva Mukha tones and strengthens the muscles of the arms and shoulder. Since it is a mild backbend, it improves circulation throughout the body and creates a sense of invigoration and energy.

Muscles involved in this pose include the erector spinae along the spine, engaged to lift and lengthen the back. The chest muscles, like the pectoralis major, and the shoulder muscles like the deltoids, are also activated. In the arms, particularly the triceps are engaged.

Adho Mukha Svanasana or Downward-Facing Dog Pose, is a fundamental pose. In this variation, using a chair, it looks different from the traditional pose but offers similar benefits. It provides a full body stretch strengthening and lengthening muscles from the arms and shoulders to the calves and ankles. Also, this variation improves flexibility in the spine, hamstrings, and shoulders, relieving tensions in the back and potentially alleviating fatigue and headaches. The inverted position of Adho Mukha can have a calming effect on the nervous system, helping reduce stress.

Muscles engaged in this pose include deltoids and other shoulder muscles, as well as the triceps, which are active in supporting the body weight. The muscles along the spine, including the erector spinae, are engaged to maintain the length of the spine. Additionally, muscles in the hands and wrist are engaged as they support the weight of the upper body.

The Urdhva Mukha-Adho Mukha sequence is done in a flowing manner. Inhale, during Urdhva Mukha and exhale during Adho Mukha, creating a smooth and rhythmic practice.

33. HIGH LUNGE-UTTHITA TRIKONASANA-VIRABHADRASANA II (2ND SIDE)

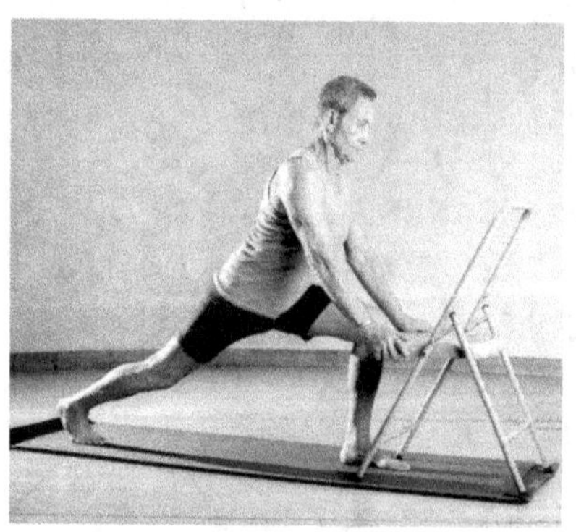
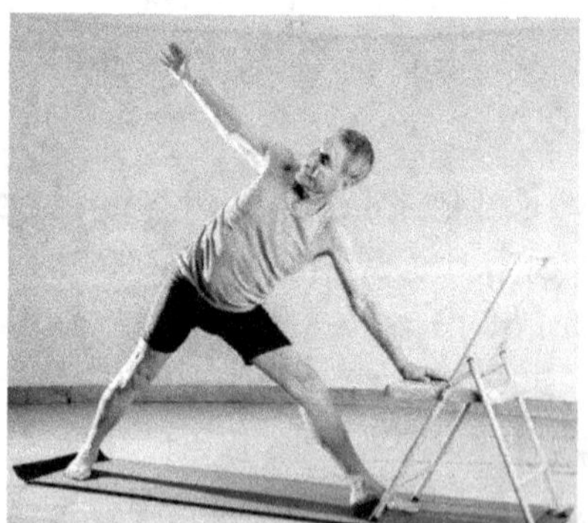

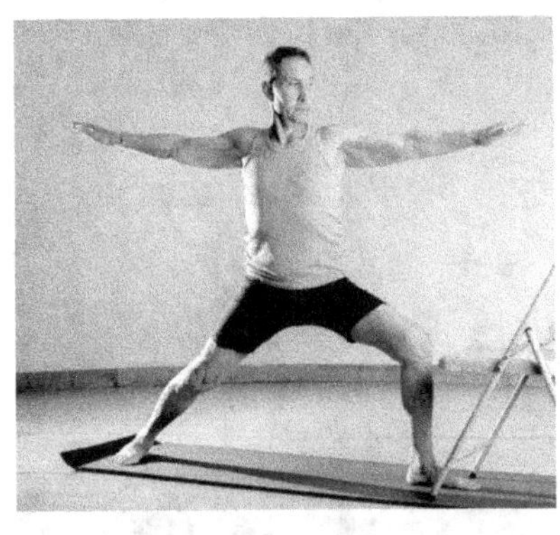
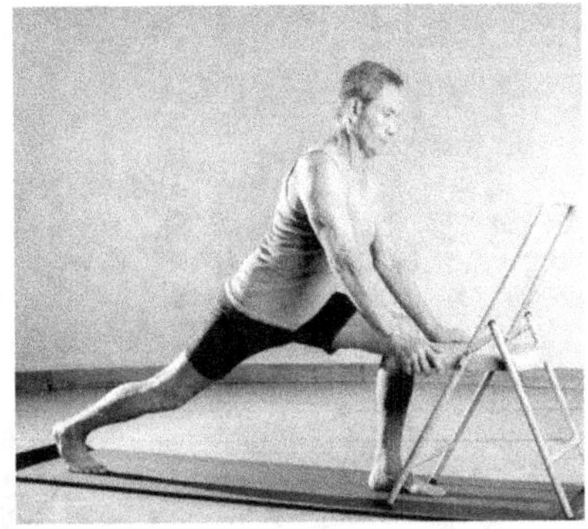

Same as the one we did before.

34. PUSH UPS-2 (10-25 Reps) – URHVAMUKHA-ADHOMUKHA

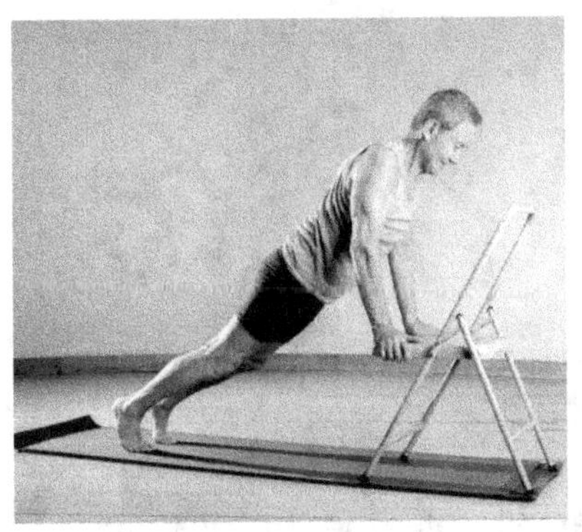
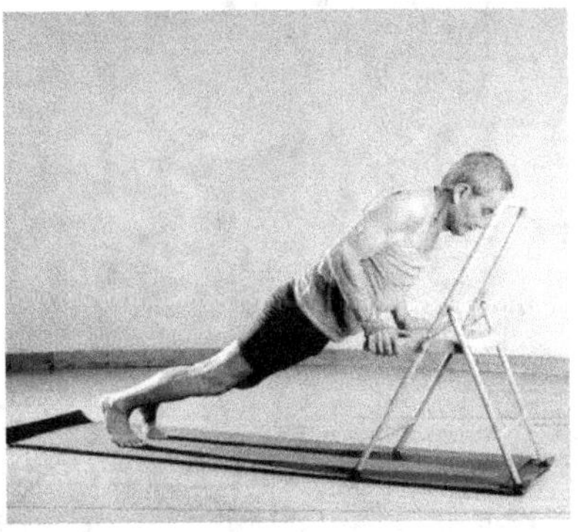

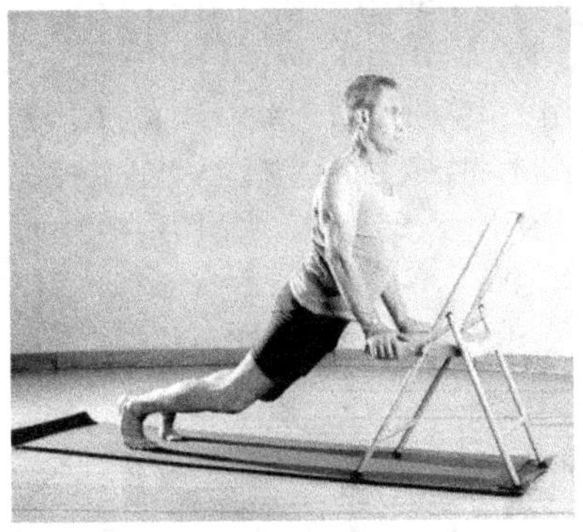
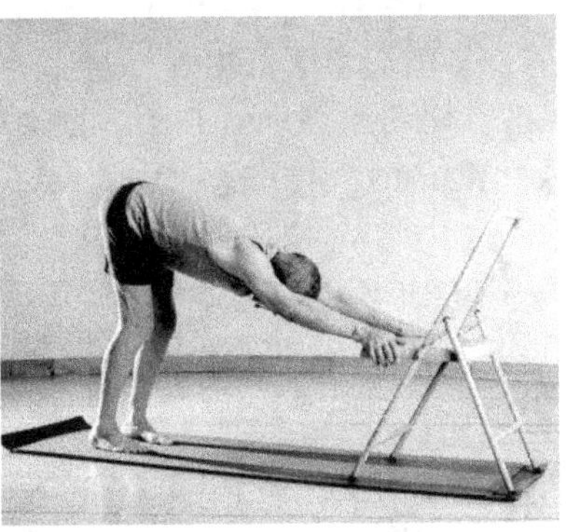

Same as the previous one.

35. HIGH LUNGE-VIRABHADRASANA I – ARROW (1ST SIDE)

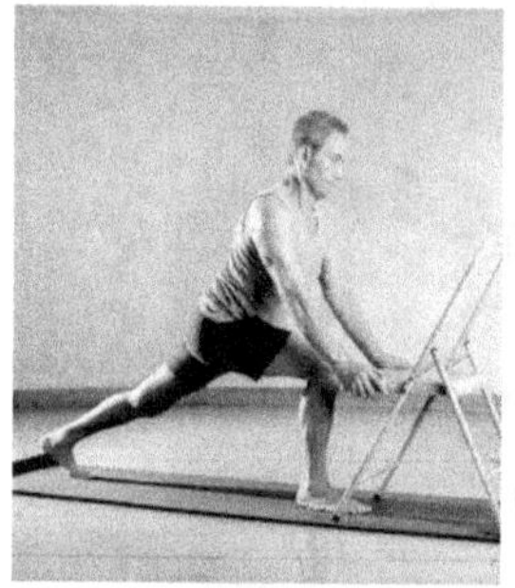

High Lunge

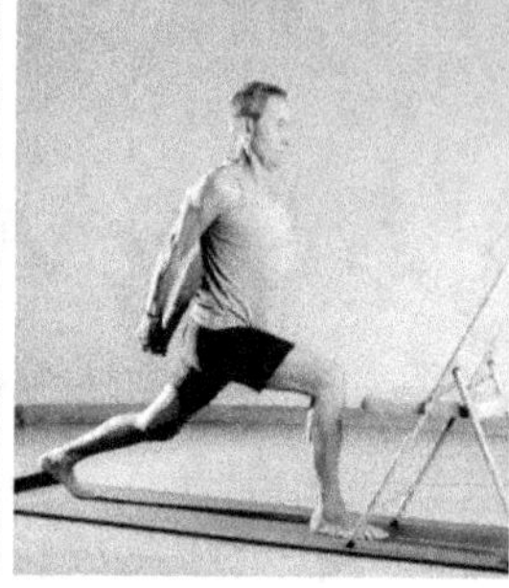

Transition

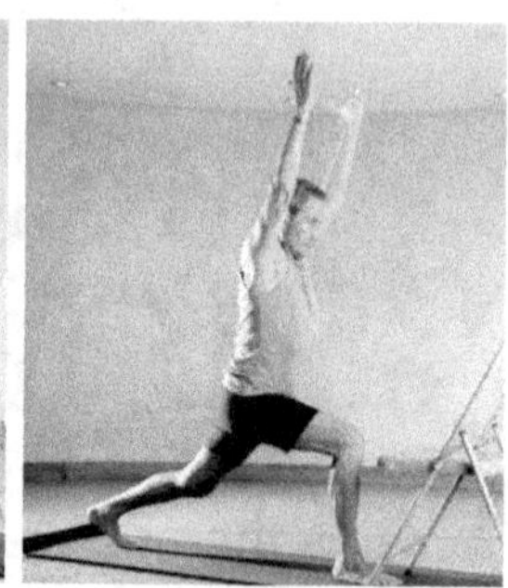

Virabhadrasana I

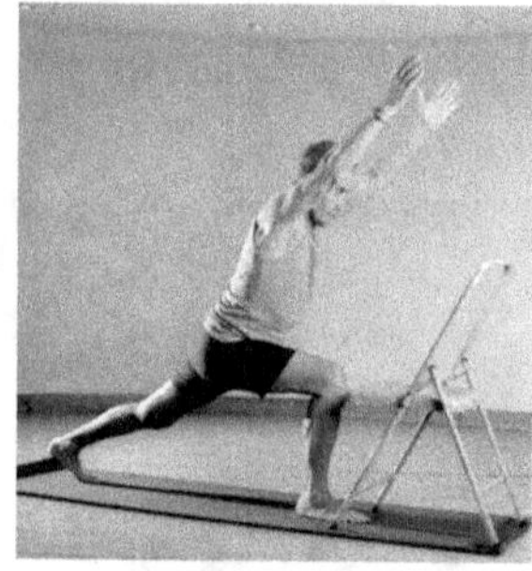

Arrow

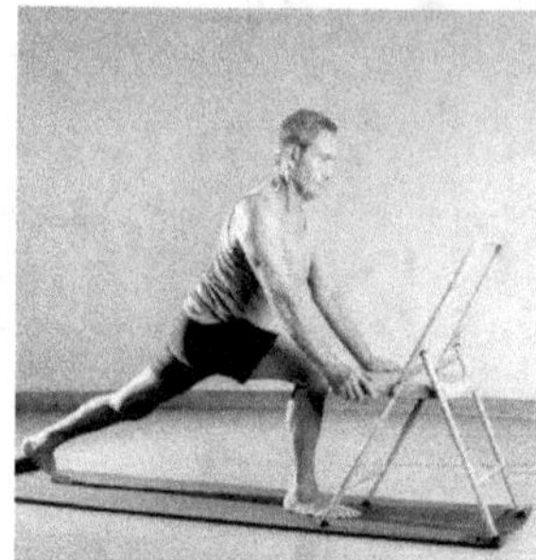

High Lunge

Now let´s explore the importance of two key standing poses in our sequence: Virabhadrasana I and "Arrow" pose. These poses play a fundamental role in our practice. To begin, we start with the High Lunge, similar to what we did in Trikonasana. Next, we smoothy transition by interlacing our fingers behind the back and straightening the torso, maintaining the leg position. This transition is a posture in its own, opening the chest and preparing us for Virabhadrasana I. After holding this pose for as long as possible, we gently incline the trunk and arms to create the shape of an "Arrow" with our bodies, while keeping the leg position intact.

Virabhadrasana I, also known as Warrior I, is a fantastic pose with benefits for your body and mind. This pose helps boost overall strength, flexibility, and mental focus. It´s especially great for improving balance and strengthening your legs, including the quadriceps, hamstrings, and calf muscles. Holding this pose for an extended period can enhance endurance and stamina. The pose also encourages concentration, aiding in the development of mental focus.

In addition to working the quadriceps and hamstrings, Warrior I engages the psoas muscles and hip flexors. These muscles deep, and at the front of the hip, are stretched when the back leg is extended. This adds to the pose´s impact on your body, promoting flexibility and strength.

The "Arrow" pose is the last one in this sequence, following Virabhadrasana I, and offers similar benefits. In both "Arrow" poses and Virabhadrasana I in this routine, the back leg heel lifted. Unlike the traditional pose where the heel is on the ground, having the back heel lifted challenges balance and allows for a better stretch in the back leg. This lifted heel also helps align the hips, which is not the case in the traditional pose. The "Arrow" posture engages the muscles of the back and the legs differently than Virabhadrasana I. While holding the pose for an extended period may be challenging, it´s recommended to stay in it for as long as possible to reap its overall benefits.

36. PURVOTTANASANA-1 (10 Reps)

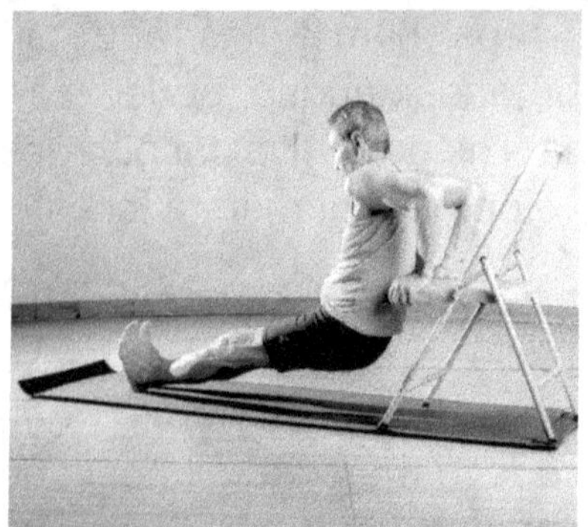 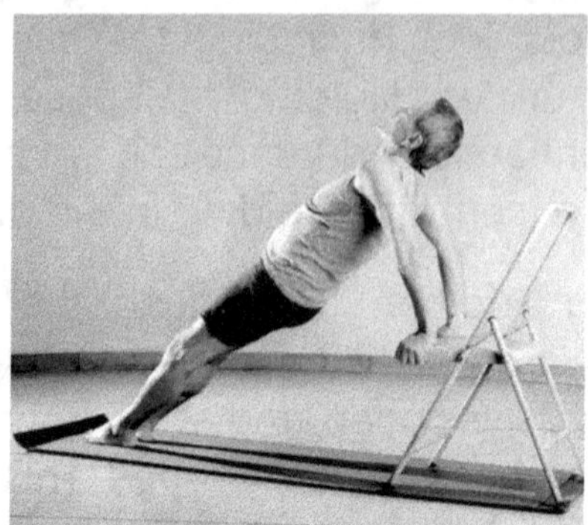

Purvottanasana

In yoga terms, what we practice here is "Purvottanasana", also known as Upward Plank Pose, a fantastic pose that involves lifting the entire body, creating a reverse tabletop position that stretches and tones the whole body, particularly the back, shoulders and core muscles.

We repeat this exercise -Purvottanasana- twice in our routine. We focus on the back of the arms, specifically the triceps muscles, which are responsible for extending the elbow join. These muscles play a crucial role when pushing or straightening your arms.

During the exercise, as you lower your body towards the floor and then push back up while holding onto the chair, the triceps are actively engaged in extending, providing essential support to the movement. This routine is excellent for strengthening your triceps.

Additionally, the triceps also play a secondary role in supporting the shoulders during specific movements, like overhead triceps extensions, contributing to stabilizing the shoulder joints.

37. HIGH LUNGE-VIRABHADRASANA I – ARROW (2ND SIDE)

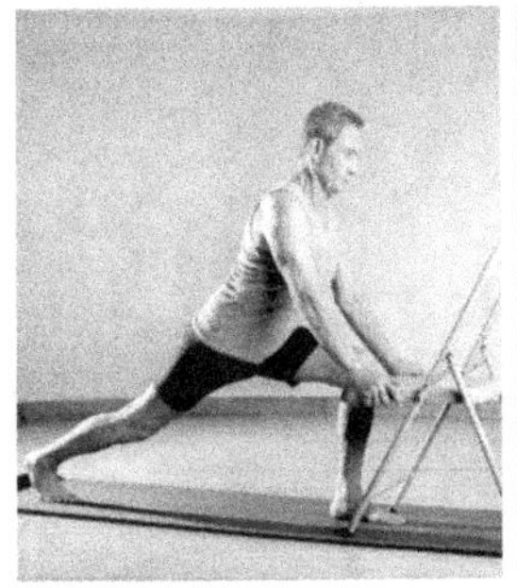 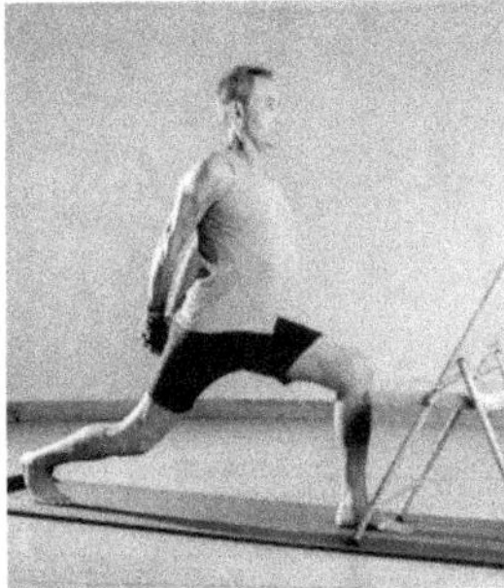 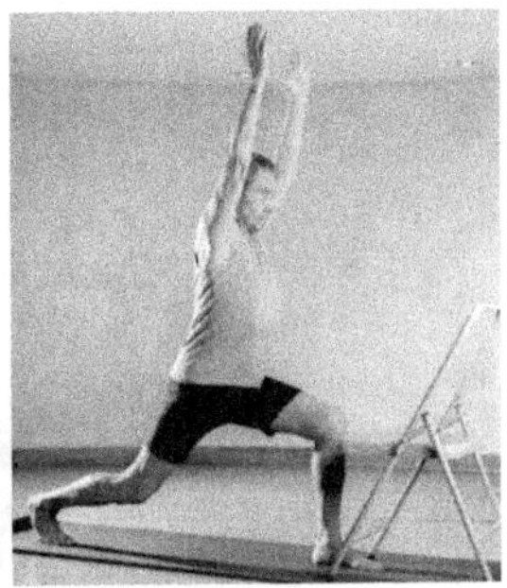

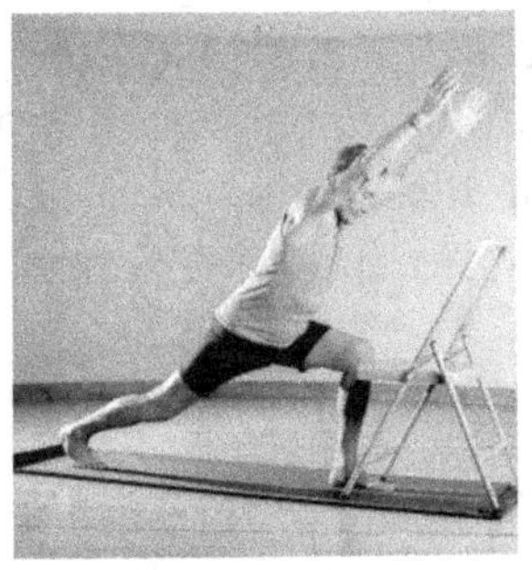 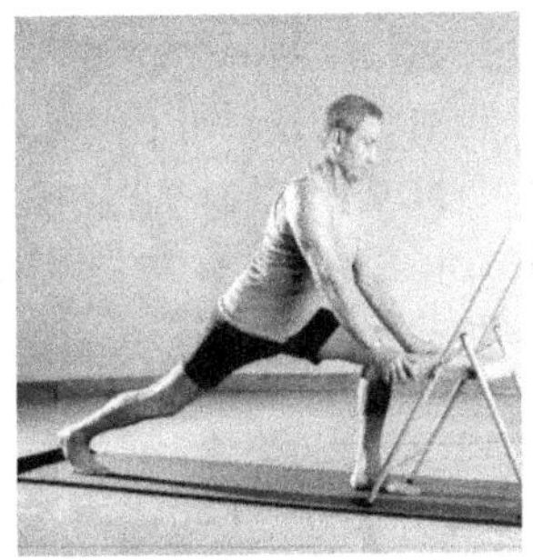

Same as the previous side.

38. PURVOTTANASANA-2 (10 Reps)

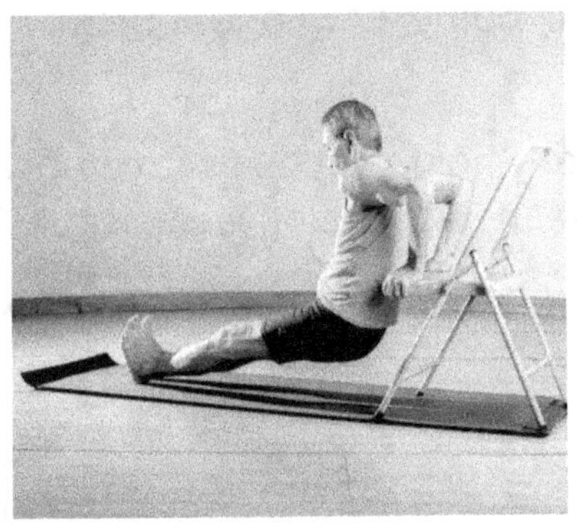 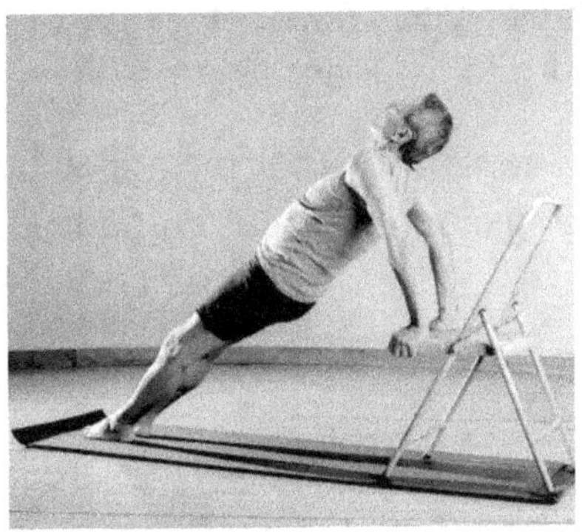

This is the second repetition of the same exercise we did before.

39. UTKATASANA (10 Reps)

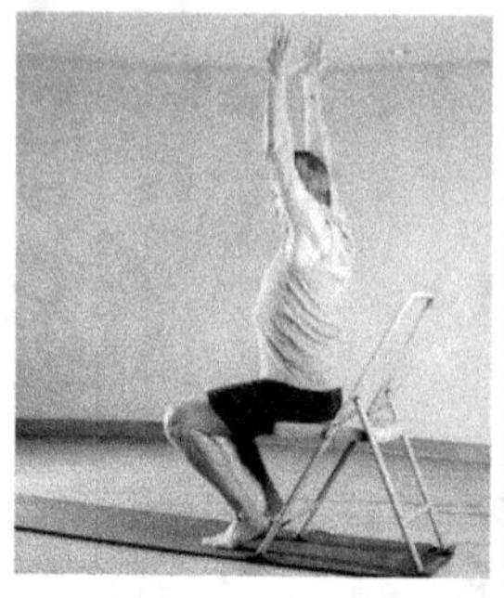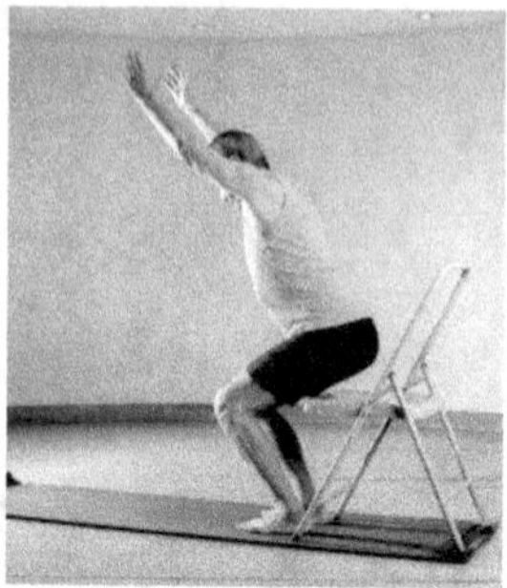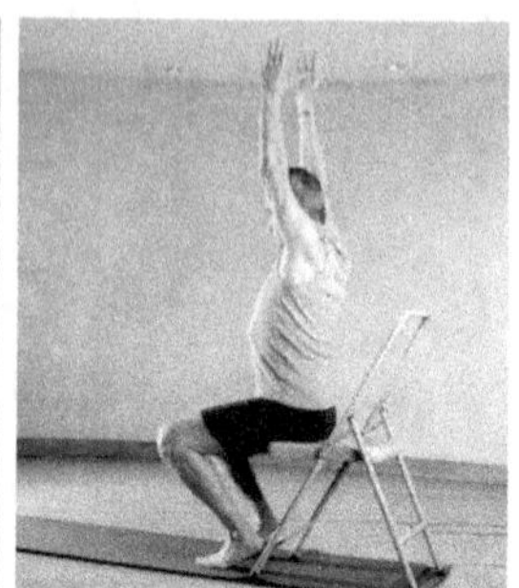

Utkatasana, commonly referred to as Chair Pose or Fierce Pose, is a powerful pose that simultaneously strengthen the lower body while enhancing posture and balance. The pose predominantly targets the muscles in the legs, core, and lower back.

To practice Ukatasana, start by sitting on the edge of the chair with arms hanging by your sides. Shift your feet back, ensuring your heels are lifted off the ground. Inhale while lifting your arms, and as you lean forward, exhale, slightly elevating your buttocks off the chair and allowing your heels to descend. Inhale again to return to the seated position, with your arms stretched toward the ceiling. As you exhale, lower your hands to your sides, completing one repetition. Aim for at least 10 reps.

When lifting your buttocks, briefly hold the pose with empty lungs, and maintaining a neutral neck position is advisable.

40. HIP OPENER 1

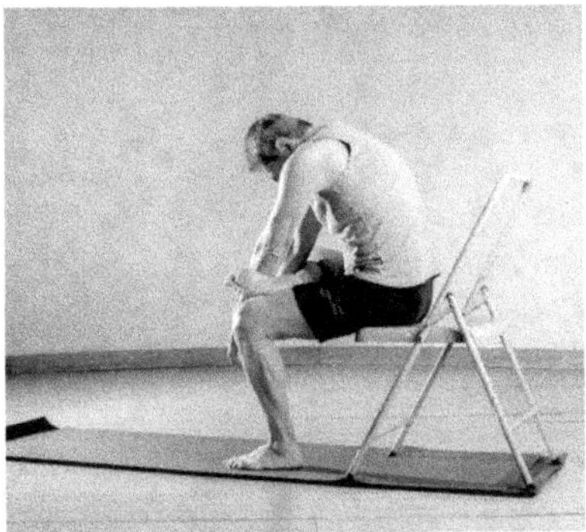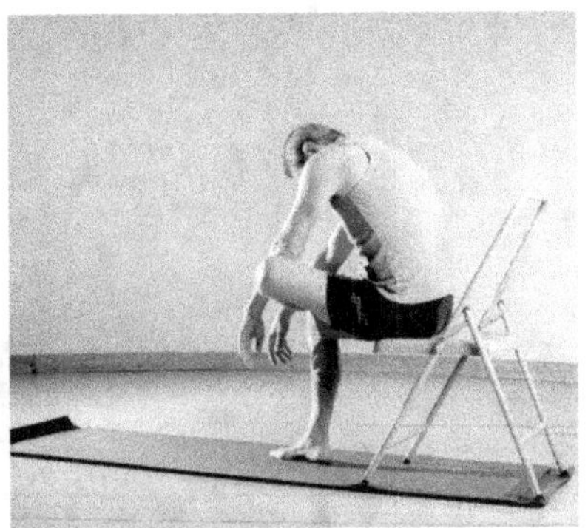

This is an easy posture than won´t take much time. Sit on the edge of the chair and place one foot on the opposite knee. Try to lower your body toward the floor. If you are flexible, (unlike me, dealing with knee issues), aim to touch the floor with your hands.

This pose is excellent for opening hip joints and stretching the spine, offering effects similar to the Pigeon Pose, also known as Eka Pada Rajakapotasana. It deeply stretches the hip flexors and increases flexibility in the hip joint, while also releases tension in the lower back.

Additionally, this first hip opener can help alleviate discomfort associated with sciatic nerve pain by stretching and releasing tension in the piriformis muscle. Moreover, it engages and stretches the gluteus maximus, the large muscle of the buttocks.

41. HIP OPENER-2

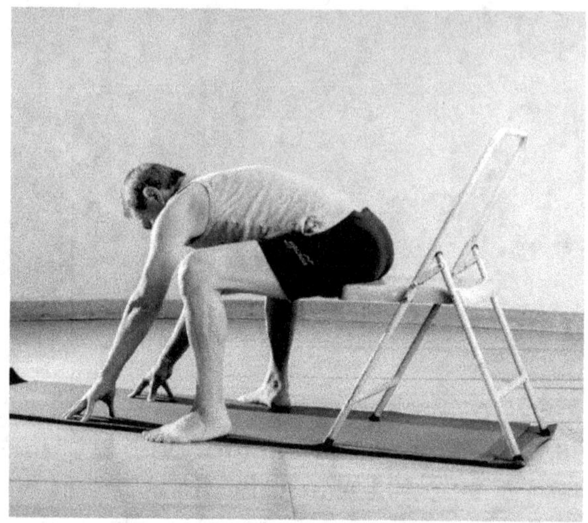

This pose is easy to do. Sit at the edge of the chair, on your sitting bones. Separate your legs and place your hands on the floor in front of you. If you can, reach forward as much as possible. This helps open your hips and stretch your spine. It is a great stretch!

42. TWIST-3

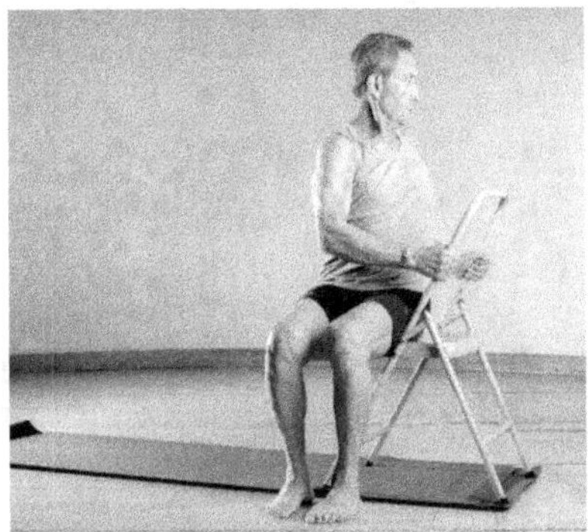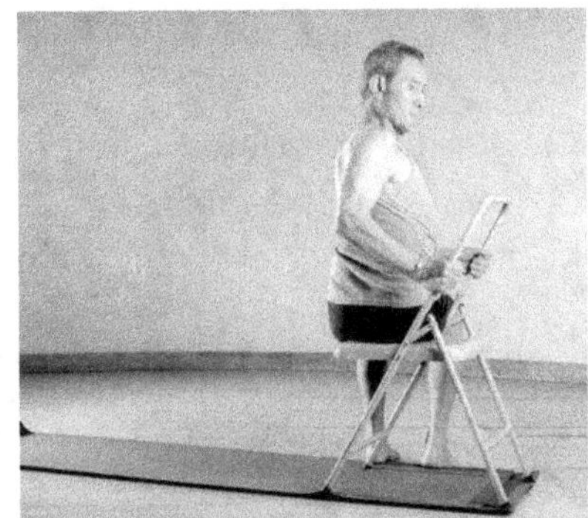

This is the final pose in this section. After lifting your upper body in the last pose, sit on the side of the chair and use your hands to grip the sides of the chair´s backrest. Twist your body in the opposite direction of your legs. Be mindful of the leg closer to the back of the chair, as it may shorten while you twist. Repeat on the other side. Remember the benefits of twisting we´ve discussed in earlier sections -they apply here too.

SIXTH SECTION: RELEASING THE SHOULDERS

This section is optional. If your shoulders are already flexible, you can skip these exercises. But if, like me, you have stiff shoulders, I recommend trying these three exercises.

Flexible shoulders are important for overall well-being and functionality. They help you have a wider range of motion in your arms and upper body, making it easier to do everyday activities and reach things. Flexible shoulders are also less likely to get strained or injured. Plus, they support good posture, reducing the risk of discomfort or muscle imbalances. Lastly, flexible shoulders can help relax the muscles in the neck, upper back, and shoulders.

43. KNEES ON THE GROUND AND HANDS ON THE CHAIR

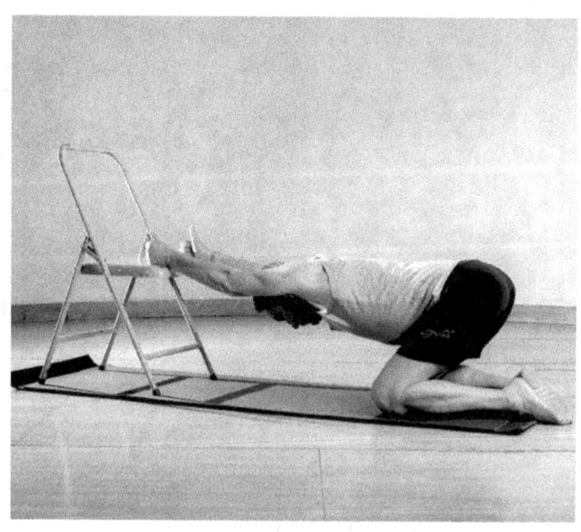

This pose works on the shoulders but also on the whole spine. To better activate the shoulder, put the thumbs up. Keep your head in between your arms. If you want, you can bring your buttocks all the way down to your heels. Holding the pose for just a few moments is enough.

44. ELBOWS ON THE CHAIR

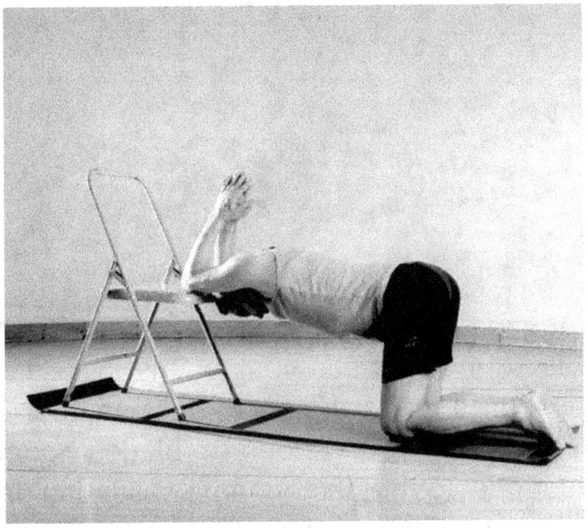

Put the elbows on the edge of the chair and join your palms. If the surface of the chair is hard, place a folded blanket on it. Align your knees with your hips. You should be able to pass your head through the space in between your elbows and your shoulders. Keep the navel in all the time. Hold this pose for a few moments.

45. RECLINING WITH PALMS RESTING ON THE CHAIR

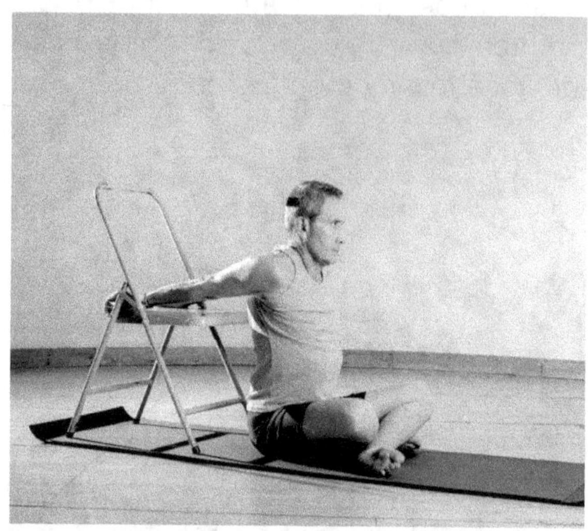

Sit cross-legged on the ground or on a folded blanket. Keep you back straight and place your palms towards the back of the chair. You´ll feel a strong rotation in your arms and shoulders, bringing your shoulder blades together and opening your chest. Stretch your spine as much as you can. When finished, take one arm at the time, carefully placing your hands on your knees. One interesting aspect of this exercise is that you´ll notice sitting effortlessly with a very straight spine.

SEVENTH SECTION: "GROUNDING"

I call this part of the routine "Grounding" because all the movements involve direct contact with the ground. This connection provides stability and a solid base, helping us work multiple muscle groups. It´s great for boosting strength, flexibility, and overall functional fitness.

46. ABDOMINALS-2 (50 REPS minimum)

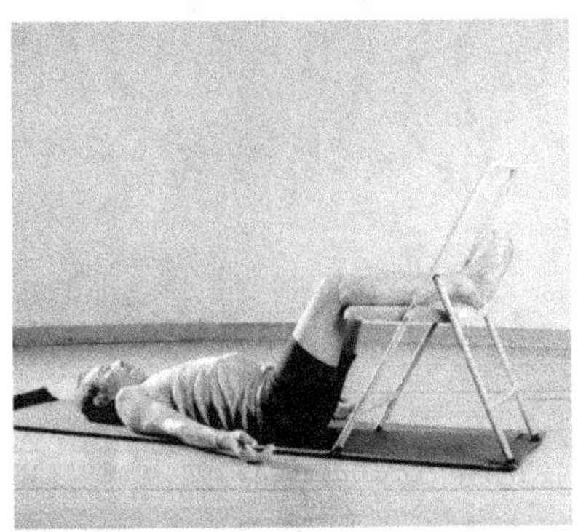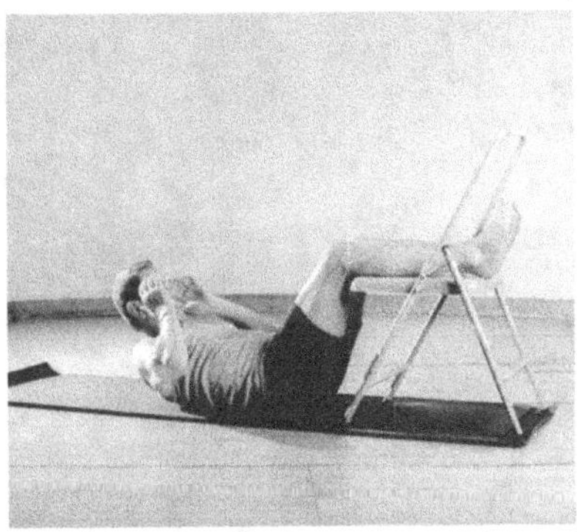

Before starting, lie on the ground with your legs comfortably resting on the chair.

Including abdominal exercises in your fitness routine is crucial for several reasons. The abdominal muscles, which consist of the rectus abdominis, transverse abdominis, and obliques, form the core. A strong core is essential for overall stability and balance, supporting movements like lifting, twisting and bending.

Strong abdominal muscles also contribute to good posture by supporting the spine and pelvis, protecting the lower back. Daily activities such as getting out of bed, picking up objects or reaching out for something involve the use of these muscles.

While is essential not to focus solely on aesthetics, many people appreciate the visual benefits of a toned core. Additionally, strong abdominal muscles provide support to internal organs, ensuring proper functioning.

Working with a chair –like in the photo– it´s not very demanding and targets both the core and the neck muscles. Place your hands on the sides of the ears, not behind the head. Aim for 50 repetitions ideally, but you can start with 25 and gradually increase.

47. PURVOTTANASANA - 3 (25 to 50 Reps)

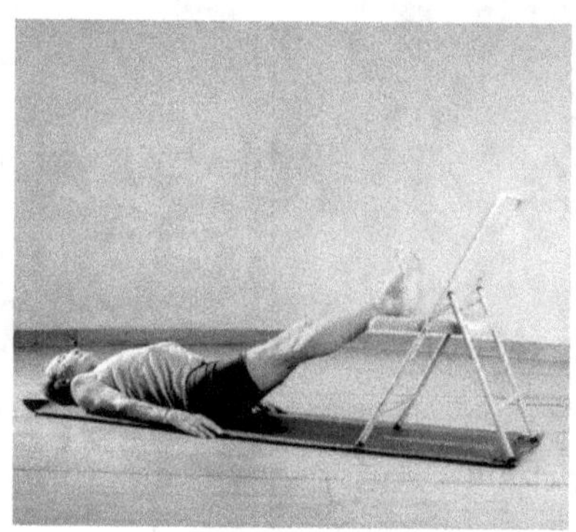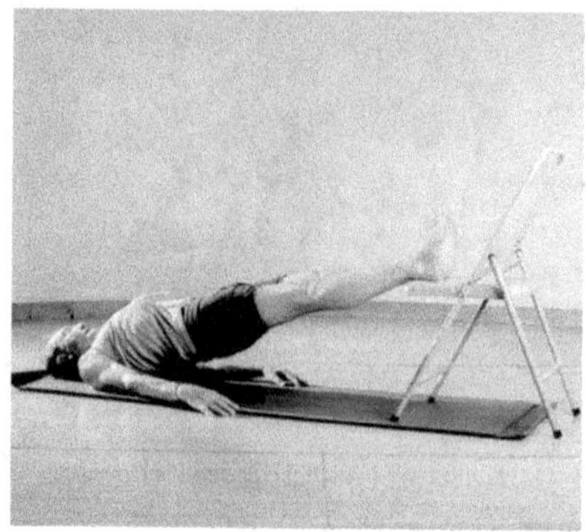

This is a variation of Purvottanasana or Upward Plank Pose. Begin by placing your heels on the edge of the chair with straight legs and your back on the floor. Keep your arms by your sides. Inhale as you lift your body, like a plank, and exhale as you lower it. Aim at least for 25 repetitions, but try to reach 50 for a more challenging workout.

48. ROLLING BACK AND FORTH

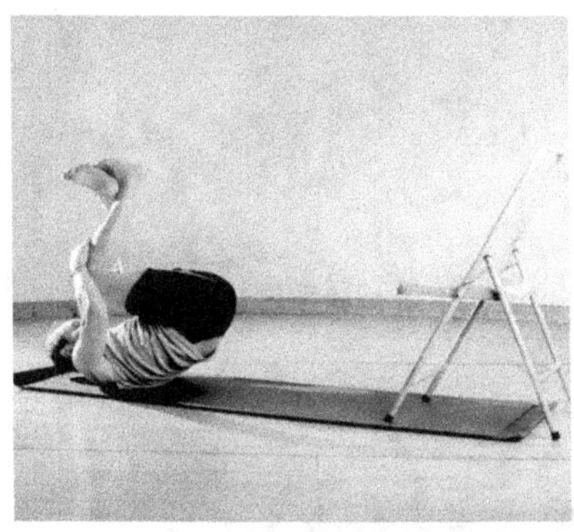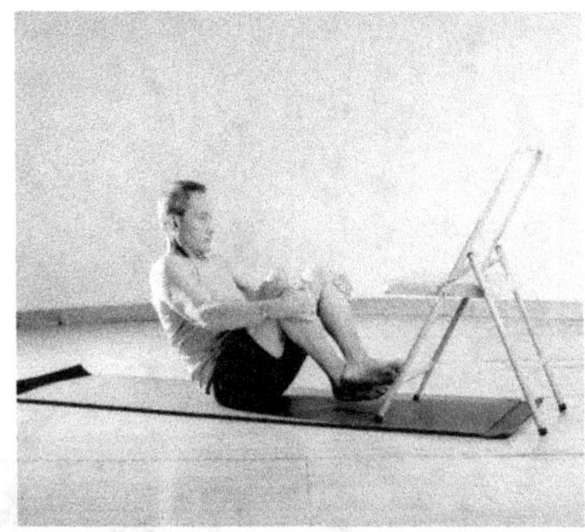

Roll back and forth, like a ball, without letting your feet touch the floor. Keep your chin close to your chest, cross your feet, and place your hands on your knees. Aim to roll seven times, and on the last roll, sit up and spread your legs for the next pose: Upavistha Konasana.

Rolling back and forth isn´t just fun – it´s beneficial for your spine. This movement acts like a mini-massage for your back and promotes better blood circulation around the vertebral discs. It´s a simple yet effective way to care for your spine and enhance its flexibility.

49. UPAVISTHA KONASANA-SANKALPA 2

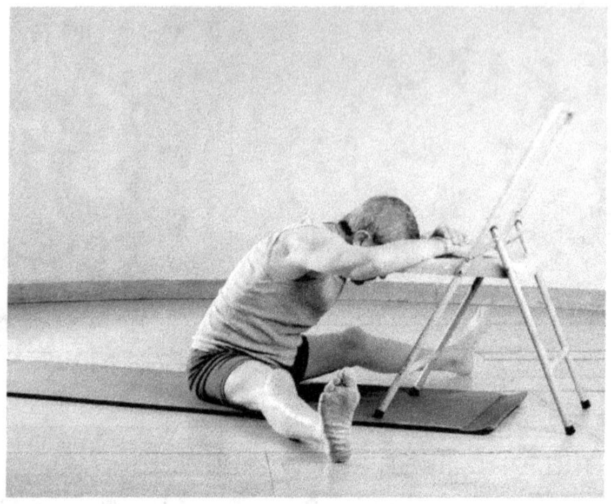

This pose, Upavistha Konasana is also known as the "Seated Wide-Legged Forward Bend". Using a chair makes it easier than the traditional pose. In Yoga for Life is considered a resting pose since the forearms and the head rest on the chair. Nevertheless, this pose contributes to opening up and stretching the inner thighs and groin, promoting flexibility in this part of our anatomy. It also engages and strengthen the muscles along the spine, promoting better posture and spinal health. The meditative nature of the pose can have a calming and soothing effect on the mind, helping to relieve stress and anxiety.

Additionally, this pose actively stretches and engages the adductor muscles located on the inner thighs. It also stretches the hamstrings, hip flexors, and the muscles along the spine, particularly the spinal extensors.

While you are in this pose, I suggest you to make your second and final Sankalpa.

50. NEO-TUMMO-PAWANMUKTASANAS AND RELAXATION

NEO-TUMMO

In my view, the essence of the Yoga for Life method, lies in what I consider its highlight -the "Neo-Tummo" technique. I´ve provided an extensive explanation of this technique in the GPBALANCE book collection, particularly in Book 4, dedicated to breathing. This technique emphasizes holding the breath after gently rocking the body back and forth, followed by a soft exhalation.

Following Upavistha Konasana, we lie on our backs, preferably in Supta Baddha Konasana. In this position, the soles of the feet are together, and the arms extend behind the head to further open the chest.

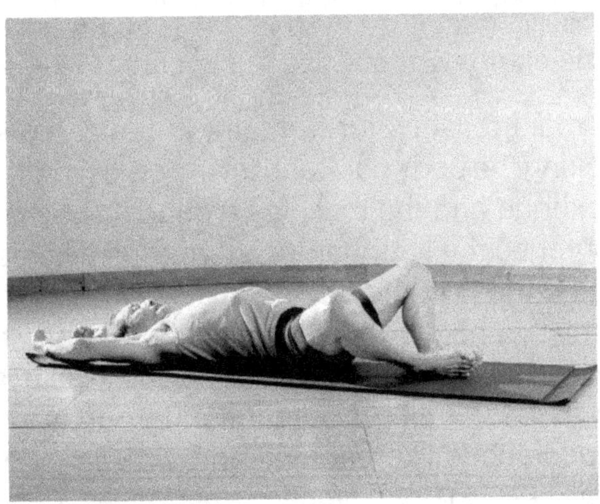

This technique is subtle and best understood by watching the video. Nevertheless, I´ll try to explain is as follows:

Firstly, lightly press the soft palate with the tongue and ensure that the pelvic floor muscles are gently contracted. Then as you inhale through the nose, softly push the body backward. This movement may not appear significant to the eyes; it´s subtle. As you complete the inhalation and relax the body, it naturally returns to the starting position with the natural exhalation. This constitutes one breath. Aim for at least 54 breaths. After the final natural exhalation, hold your breath with empty lungs for as long as you can. You might feel tingling in the arms, hands and legs. You might feel tingling in the arms, hands and legs. When the desire to breathe in is irresistibly, breath in and hold your breath on full lungs for about 10 to 15 seconds, then exhale and breathe normally once and repeat this process two more times, totaling three times. Once finished, you´re ready to proceed with the next chapter on Pawanmuktasanas.

Now, let me clarify why we use this technique:

I see two main reasons for it: firstly, it gently works on the spine. Rocking the body back and forth acts as a soft massage to the backbone and the muscles around it. This movement also encourages the lymphatic system, which is responsible for balancing fluids in the body and supporting the immune system. The lymphatic system contains a clear fluid with white blood cells that help eliminate toxins, waste, and extra fluid from tissues. It´s crucial for filtering out and capturing harmful substances like bacteria and viruses, boosting the body´s defenses against infections and diseases.

The second goal is to intentionally increase carbon dioxide in the blood. This deliberate elevation creates a state of hypoxia, prompting a surge in red blood cells. This process ultimately enhances oxygen levels in the body.

PAWANMUKTASANAS

It´s known as "Wind-Relieving Poses", a set of yoga exercises crafted to ease gas in the digestive system, enhance digestion, and boost flexibility in joints and limbs to release tension and increase energy flow in the body.

These exercises trace their origin to traditional Hatha Yoga and Ayurveda, handed down through generations as part of broader yogic practices. I´ve introduced some new Pawanmuktasana poses in this routine, concluding the Yoga for Life practice.

Pawanmuktasana 1

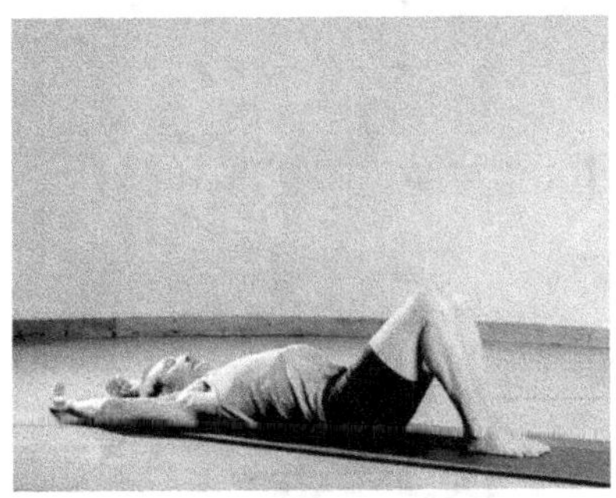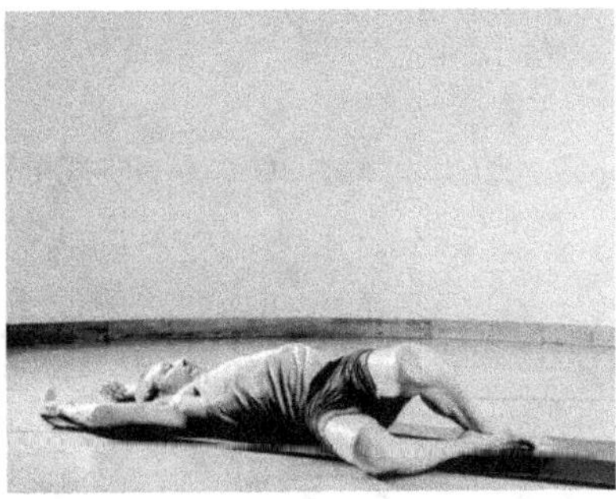

Extend your arms behind your head and keep your feet on the ground with your knees together. Exhale as you bring both legs to one side and inhale as you move them to the other side, keeping your feet on the ground. Repeat this motion at least ten times on each side. This gentle exercise provides relaxation and soothes, massaging your internal organs and muscles around your waist. Keep your eyes closed for a more serene experience.

Pawanmuktasana 2

This Pawanmuktasana is similar to the previous one, but now separate the feet to the width of the mat. You´ll feel a bit more stretch on your waist and hip joints. Repeat this movement at least ten times on each side. After finishing, lie on your left side to smoothly transition to the next exercise.

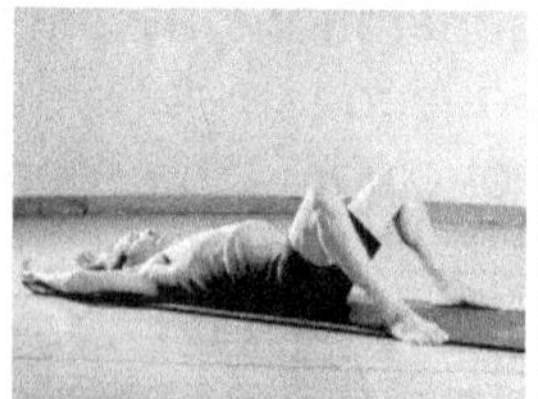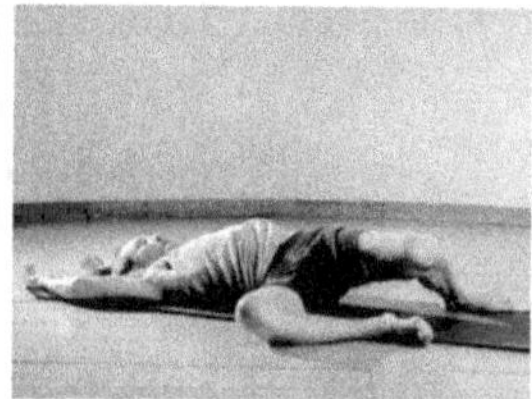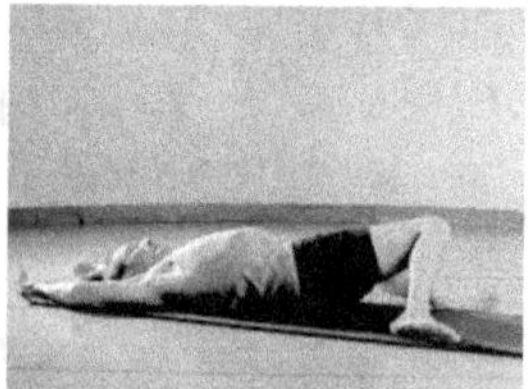

Transition

Now you are ready to start the third Pawanmuktasana:

Pawanmuktasana 3: Twist

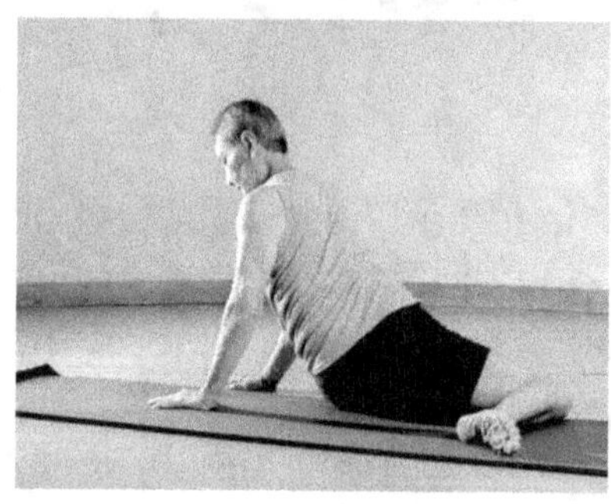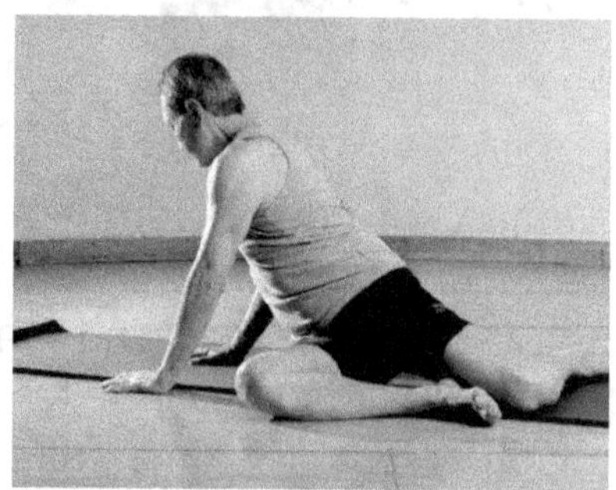

Maintain a 90-degree angle with your left thigh and align your hands with your shoulders. Keep your arms straight. You´ll feel a twist in your waist, particularly around your right kidney. Focus on your adrenal glands and practice Bhastrika 1 for 15 seconds. Repeat the exercise on the opposite side. This technique helps activate the adrenal glands, an essential element of GPBALANCE (Hormone Yoga).

Maintaining the health of the adrenal glands is crucial for overall well-being and the proper functioning of various bodily systems, like stress management, energy production, immune system support, metabolism regulation, blood pressure control, mood and emotional well-being, cognitive functions, sleep quality, blood sugar regulation and healthy skin.

Pawanmuktasana 4: Genital rubbing

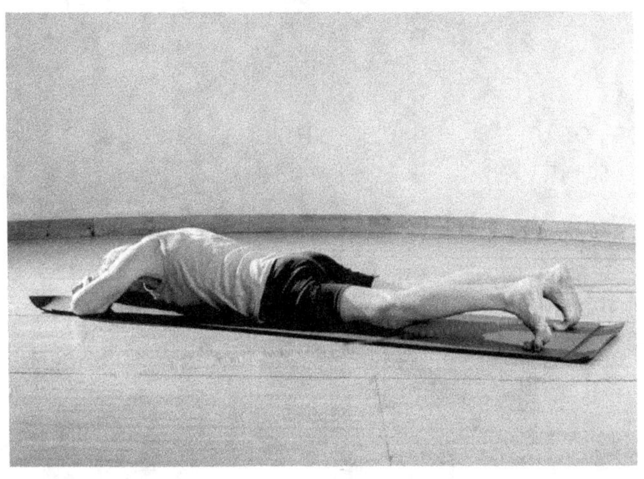

According to Master Mantak Chia, rubbing the genital area can boost sexual hormone levels and awaken the libido for both men and women. Here´s a simple exercise to try.

Lie on your stomach with your arms relaxed on the ground above the head. Using the ball of your feet, gently push your body forward, applying slight pressure to the pubic area. Let your body return to the starting point naturally. Try to synchronize this movement with your breath. Repeat this back-and-forth motion about 30 times.

Pawanmuktasana 5: Pubic tapping

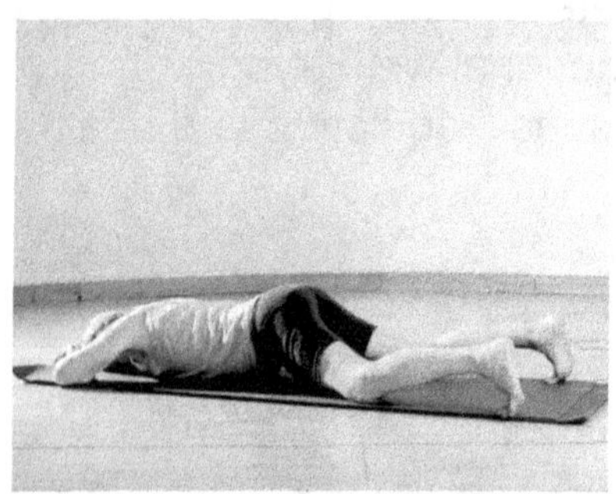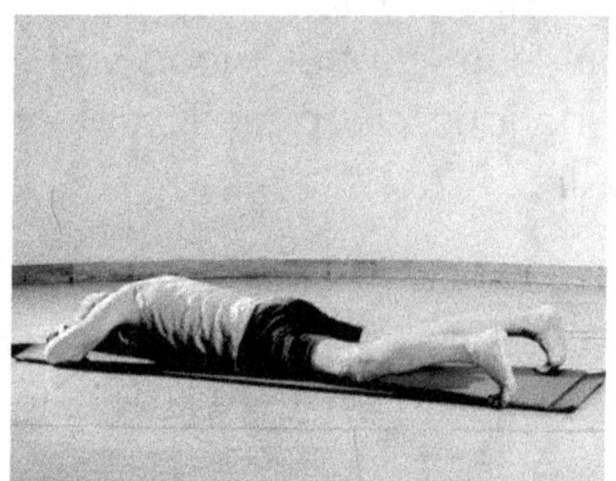

The goal of this exercise is similar to the last one. Here´s how we do it:

Stay on your stomach as in the previous exercise. Spread your feet a bit and keep firmly your knees on the ground. Inhale as you lift your hips as high as you can, then exhale and lightly tap your pubic bone on the ground. Repeat this movement at least 30 times.

Pawanmuktasana 6: Scapular girdle

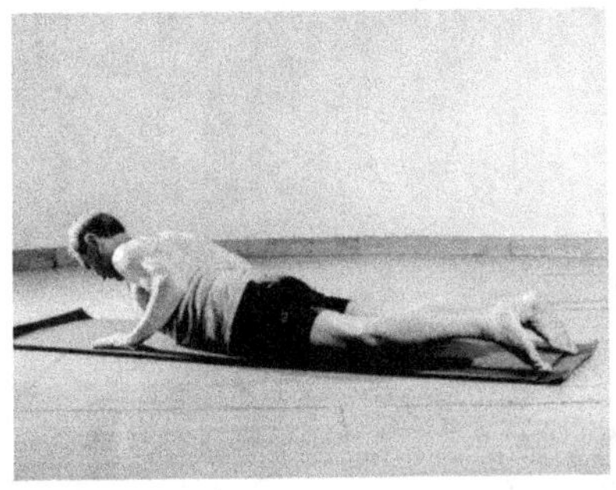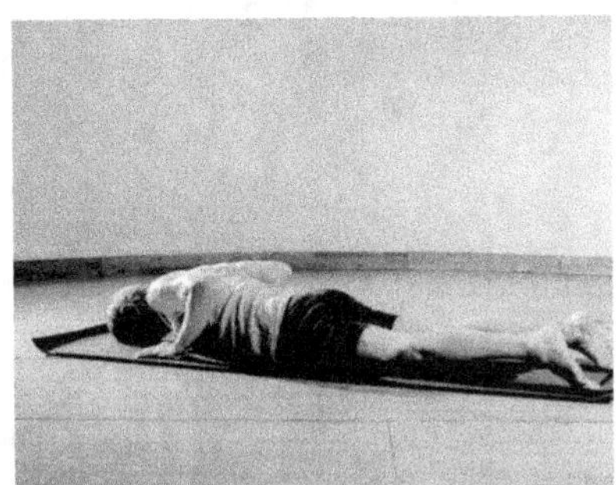

This Pawanmuktasana is part of the Shalabhasana family. The focus is on lifting the upper body without using your hands too much. Lightly press your pubic bone against the ground, and keep your legs relaxed. Try to align your head with your neck. Inhale as you lift your upper body, and exhale as you bring it back to the ground.

Shalabhasana also known as the Locust Pose, offers numerous benefits for both physical and mental well-being. Some key advantages include strengthening the back muscles, toning the leg muscles -particularly the glutes and thighs- and providing an energizing effect while stimulating the nervous system.

Pawanmuktasana 7: Knee lifting

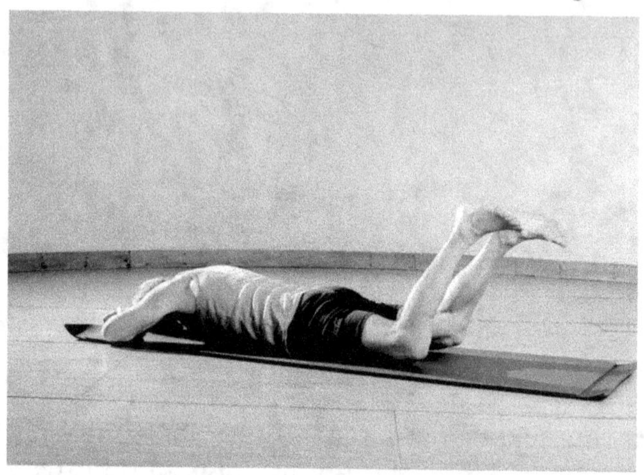

This is a unique Pawanmuktasana that originated from my creative mind. It proves effective as it encourages pressure on the pubic area and engages the pelvic floor muscles. Here´s how to do it:

Remain on your stomach, similar to the previous exercise, and attempt to lift your knees keeping your legs in a 90-degree angle. Repeat this movement ten times. Don´t be concern about your breath, as lifting the knees may temporarily affect your ability to breathe due to diaphragm engagement.

Pawanmuktasana 8: Cobra

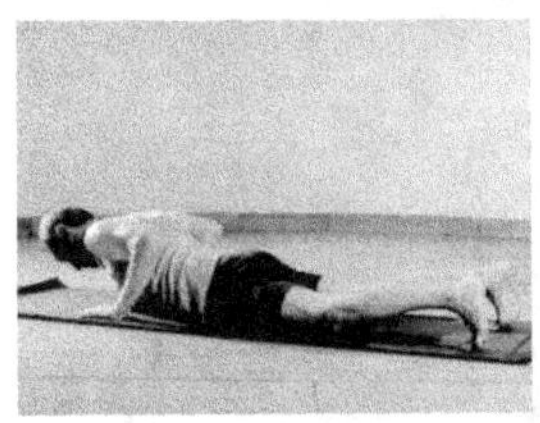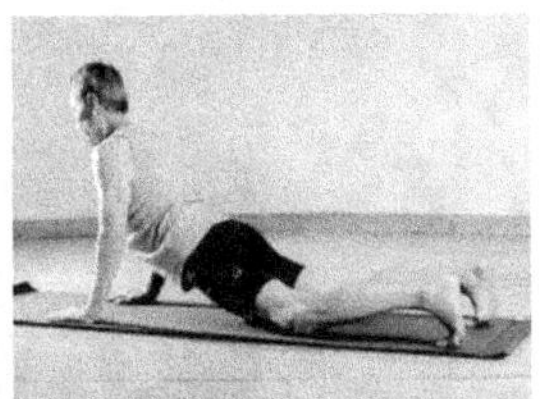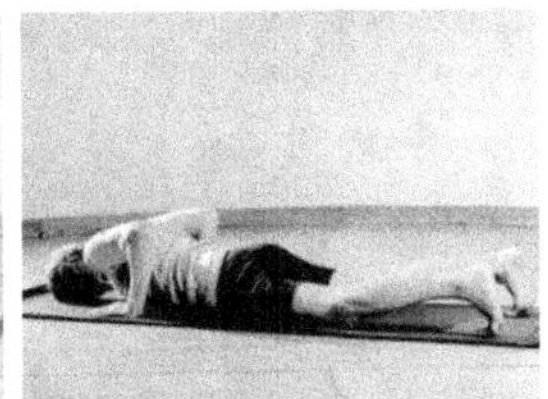

This Pawanmuktasana combines two exercises: Bhujangasana or Urdhva Mukha Svanasana (either one can be chosen) and arm bending, resembling a mild push-up. Performing Bhujangasana is generally easier than Urdhva Mukha Svanasana. In both variations, the entire body descends to the ground during the exhalation. To execute, begin by lying on your stomach with your hands positioned under the shoulders. Inhale as you extend your arms, lifting the upper body, and the exhale as you return to the floor. Repeat this sequence 10 times.

Bhujangasana, also known as Cobra Pose, provides a range of physical and mental benefits. Foremost among these is its capacity to strengthen the back muscles, with a particular focus on the lower spine. Additionally, it enhances flexibility in the spine, neck, and shoulders while toning the muscles in the buttocks and glutes. This pose is closely linked to the heart chakra (Anahata), contributing to the opening and balancing of this energy center. As a result, it nurtures emotions of love, compassion, and overall emotional well-being.

Pawanmuktasana 9: Child´s pose

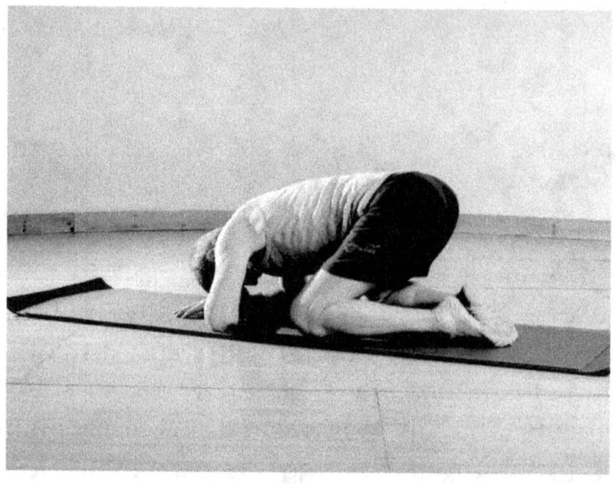

Child´s pose embodies qualities of passivity and protection, serving as a restful counterpart to the Cobra Pose in Yoga for Life. Assuming this posture provides an opportunity to engage in contractions of the pelvic floor muscles -an aspect I consider undervalued, yet crucial within our body.

Pawanmuktasana 10: Praying position

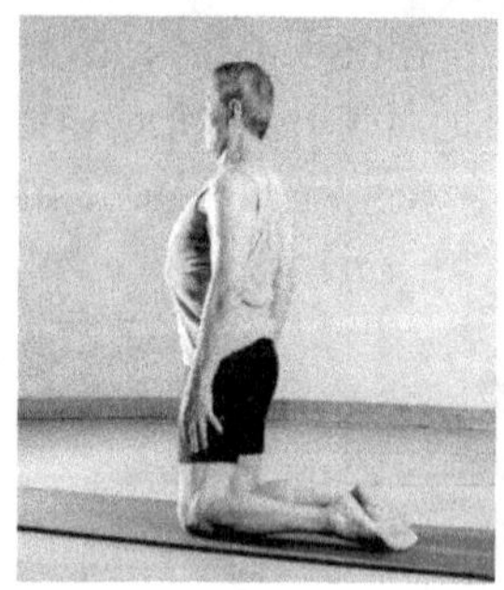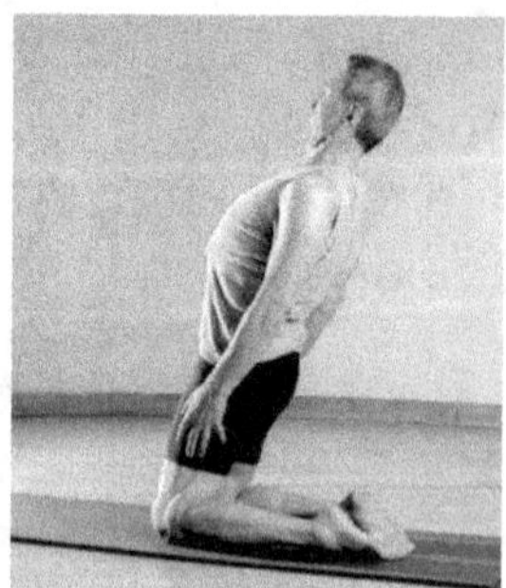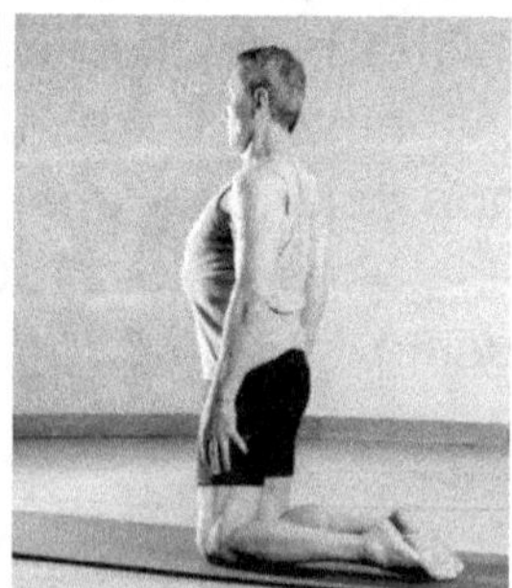

Assume the prayer position, resembling the posture you use in a church. Your arms can rest by your side, or you may choose to bring the palms together in front of your chest. Maintain alignment by keeping your head in line with the spine, forming a seamless connection with your ears, hips and knees. Engage your pelvic floor muscles, exhale as you gently lean your body backward, and inhale as you return to the starting position. Repeat this sequence 10 times.

This Pawanmuktasana not only strengthens your buttocks and legs but also serves as a transition to the next Pawanmuktasana – a mindful method of transitioning to a standing position.

Pawanmuktasana 11: Getting up

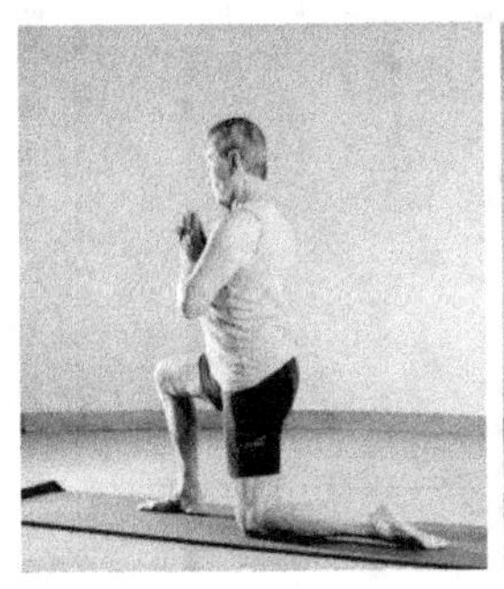
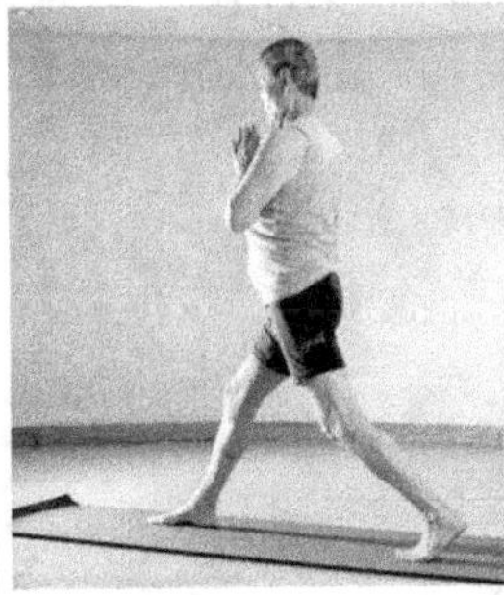
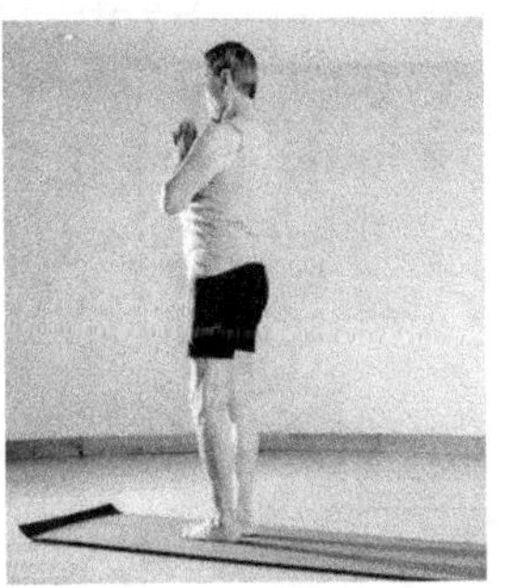

From the Prayer Pose, extend one leg outward to create a 90-degree angle, placing the ball of your back foot on the mat. Gradually and evenly press both the front and the back foot, lifting your body into a straight line. Extend your knees and bring the back foot to meet the front foot. You have now transitioned into Tadasana.

RELAXATION

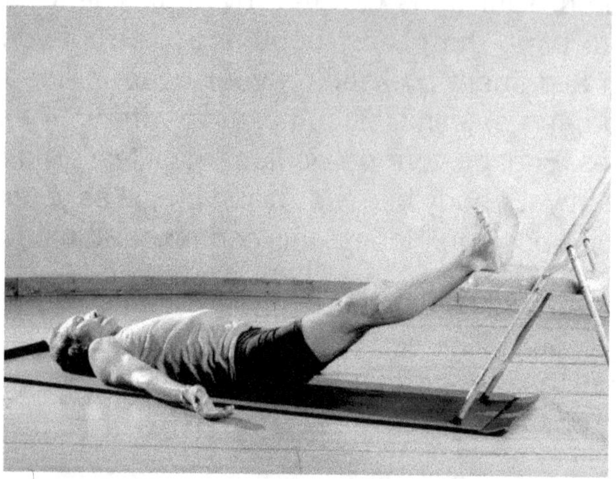

We have reached the conclusion of the Yoga for Life sequence -the relaxation. You can choose to either adopt the position with your feet on the chair or experience the tranquility of Shavasana, the Corpse Pose. Even dedicating 5 minutes to laying on your back can significantly contribute to your overall wellbeing.

PHOTO GALLERY

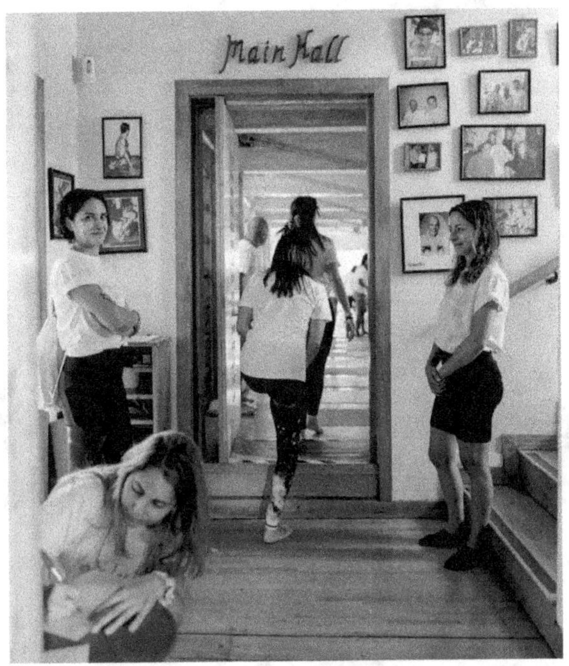

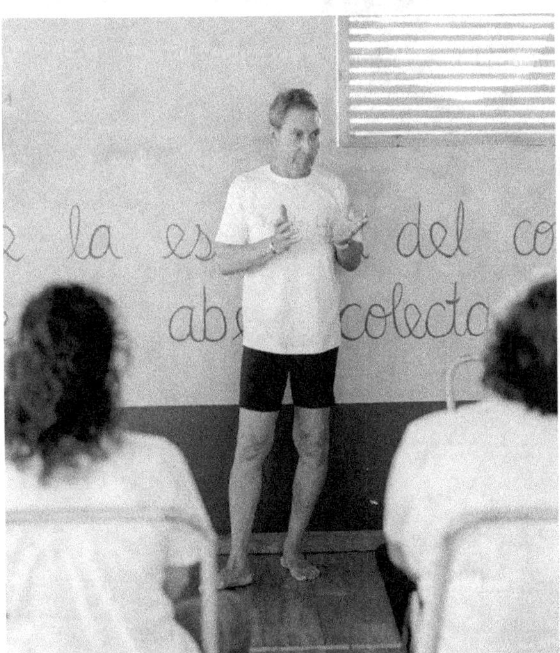

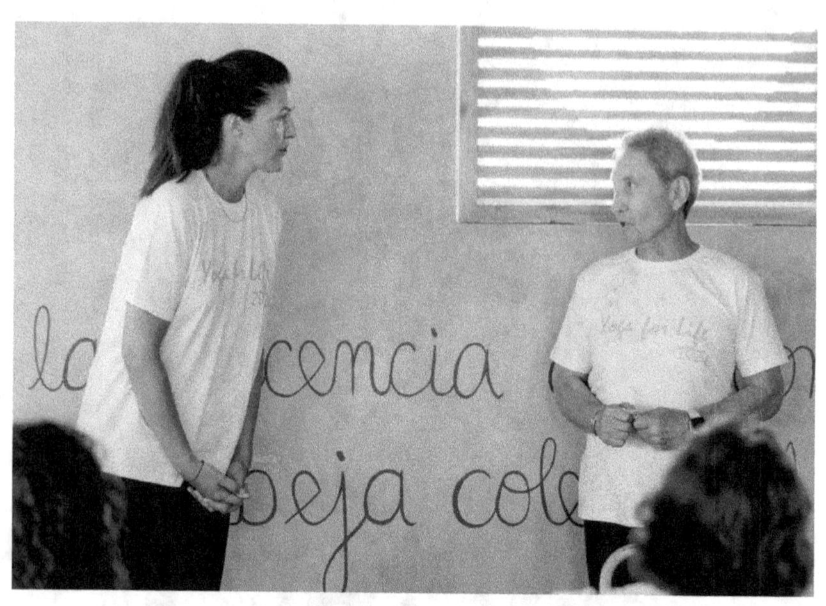

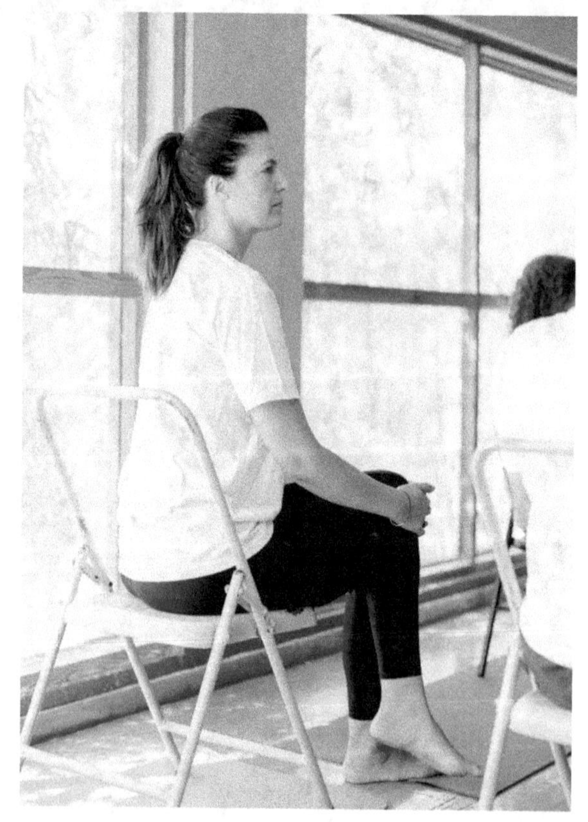

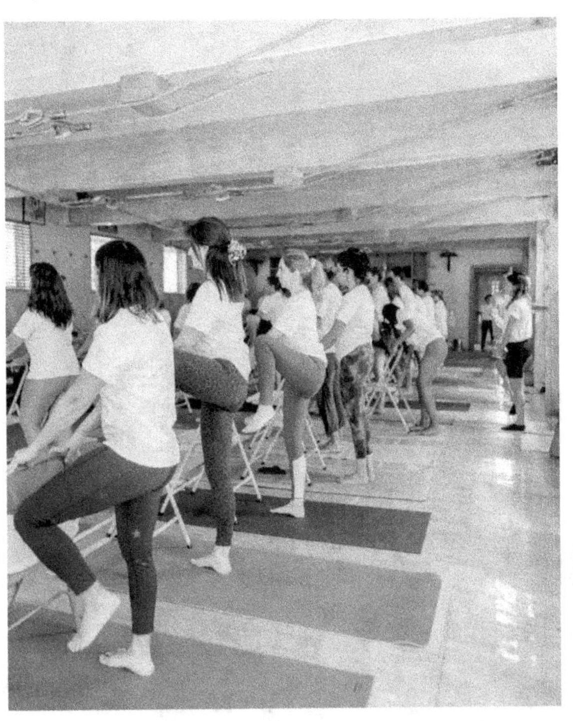

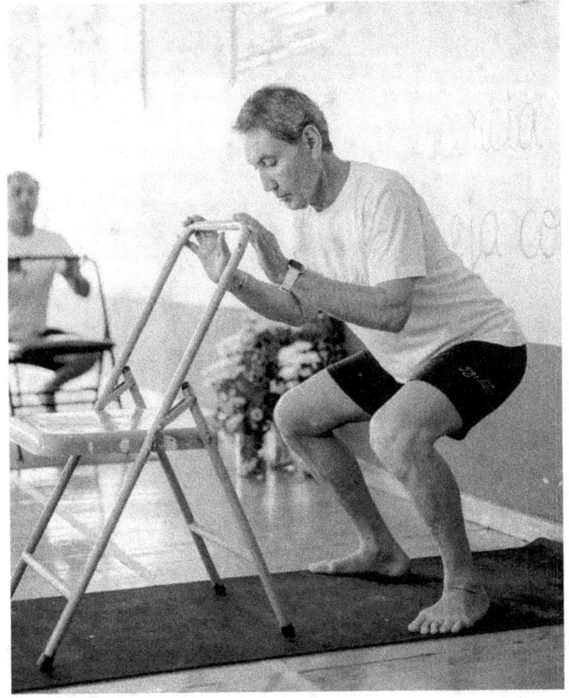

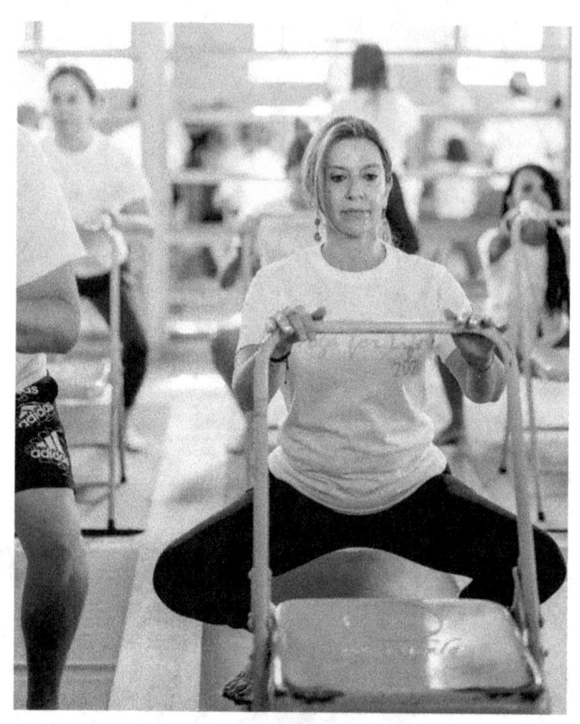

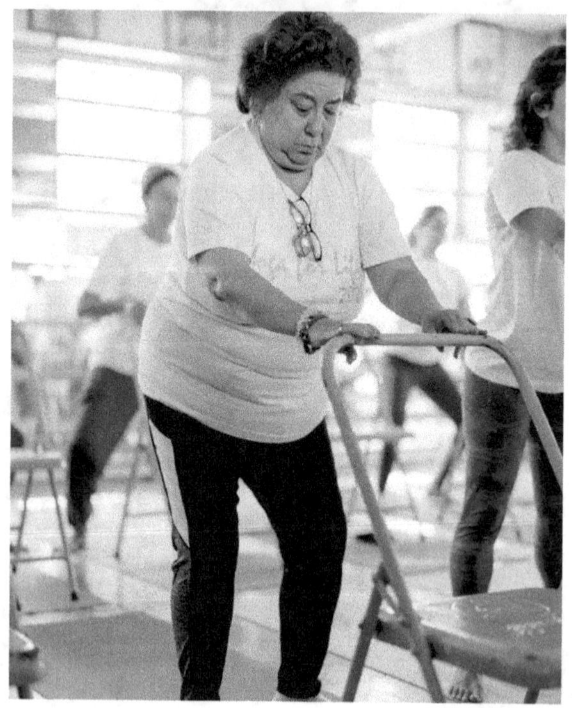

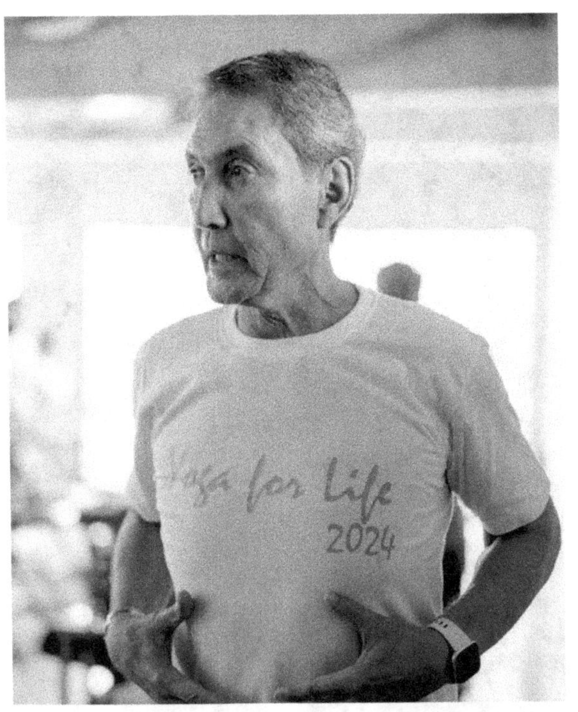

yoga for life
2024

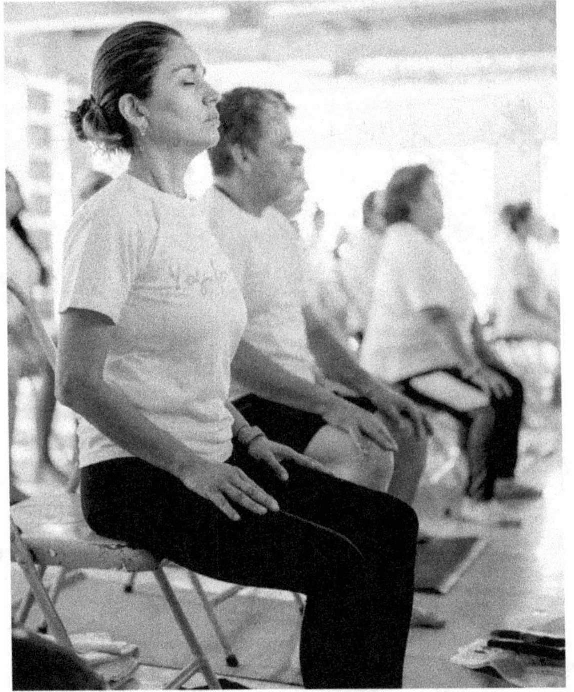

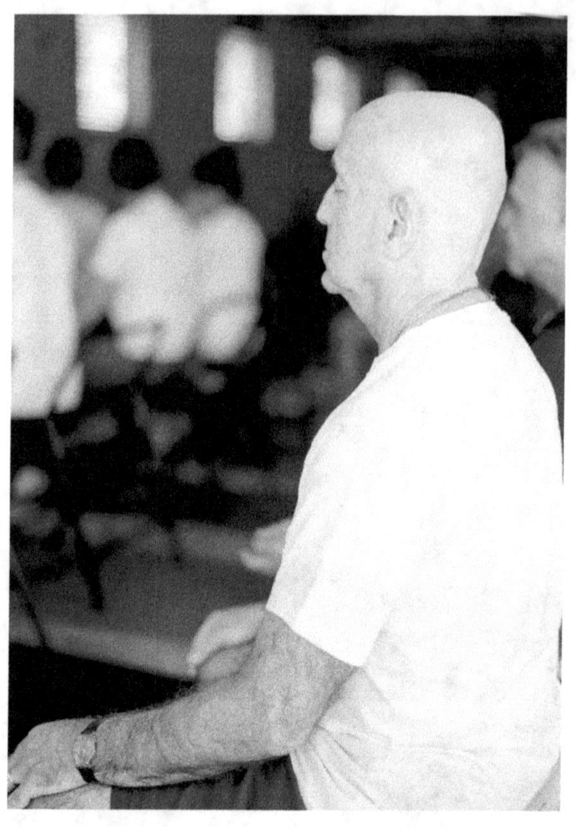

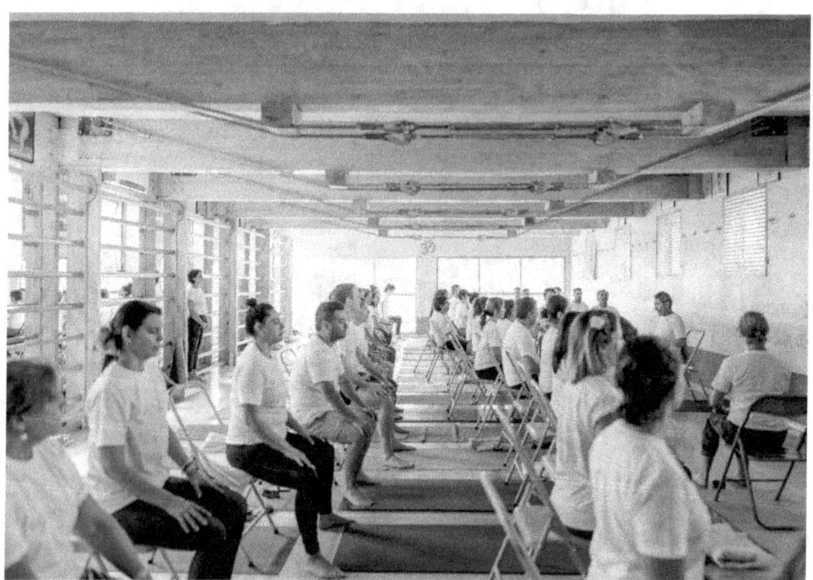

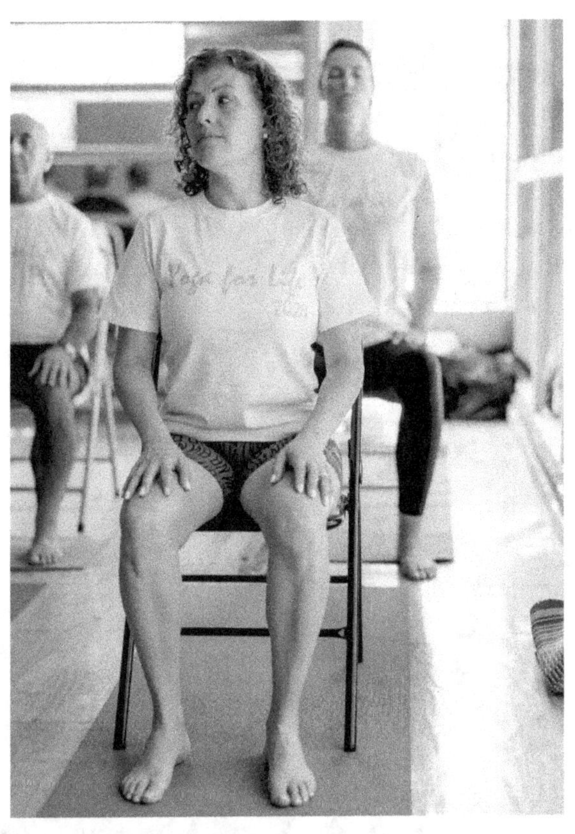

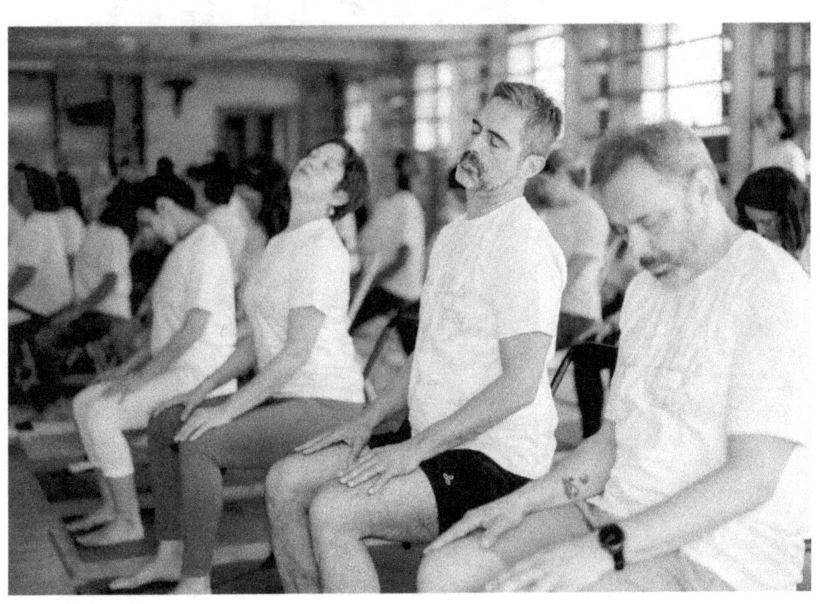

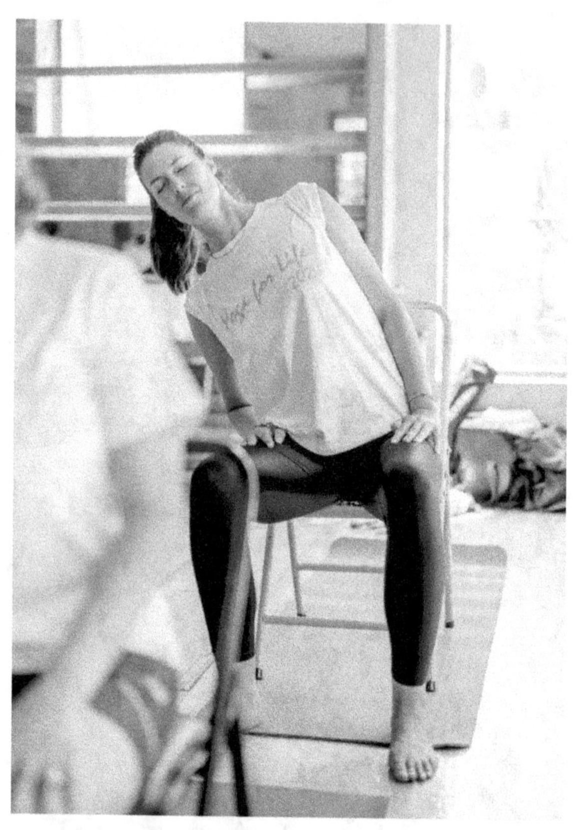

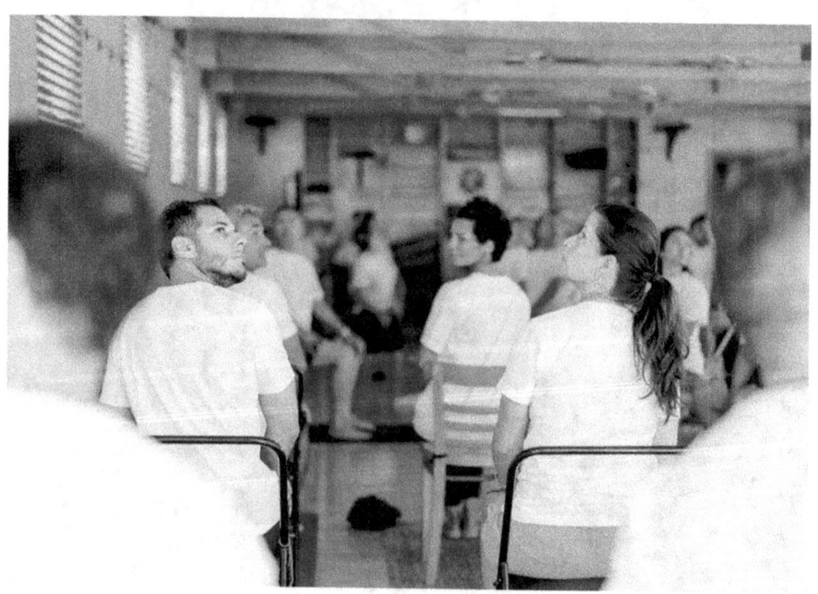

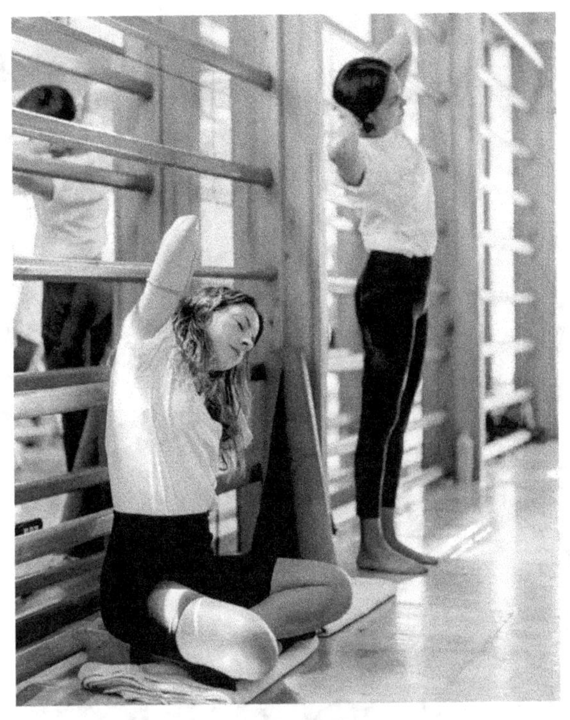

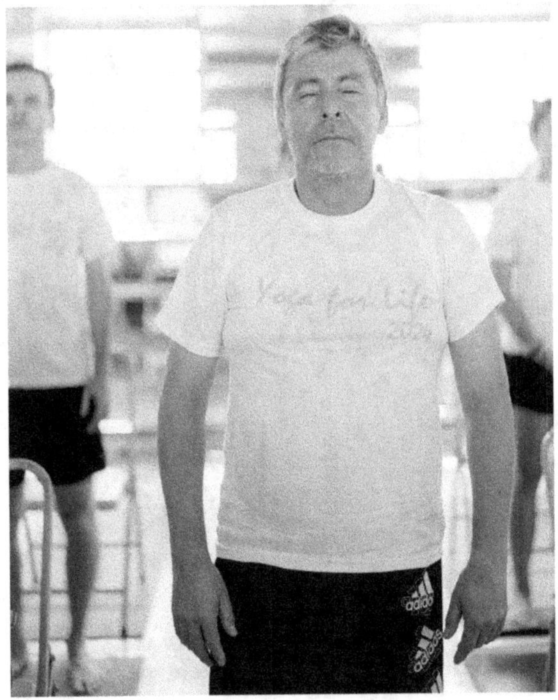

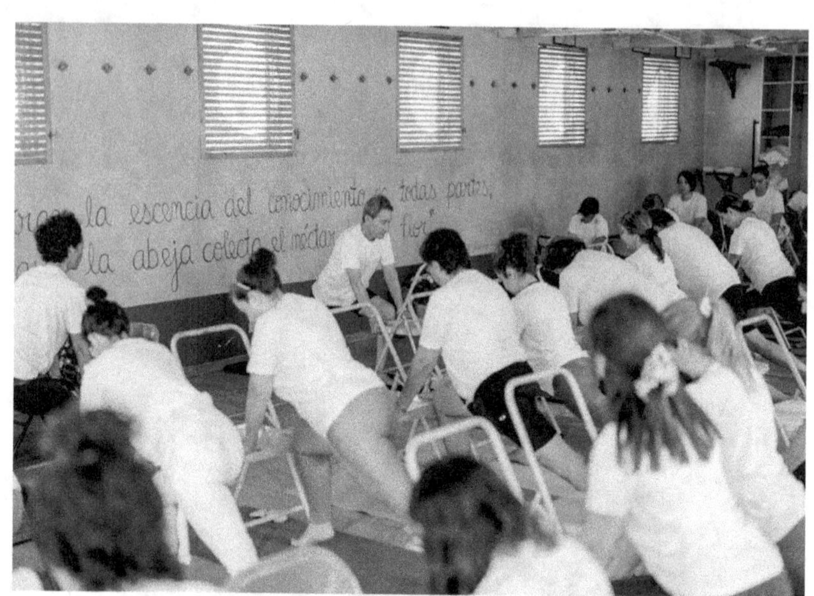

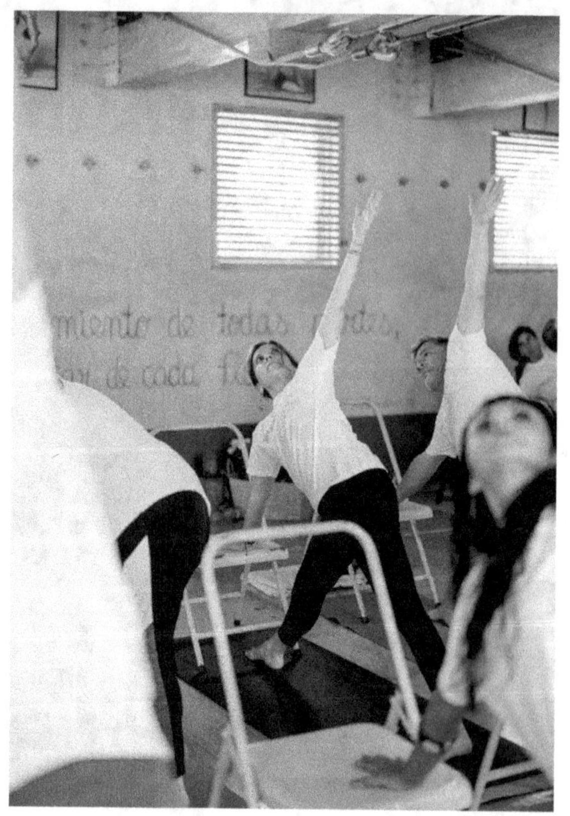

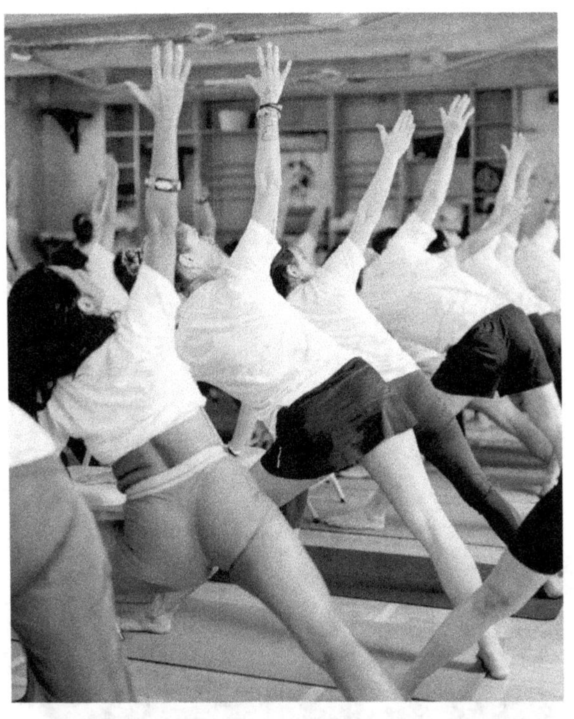

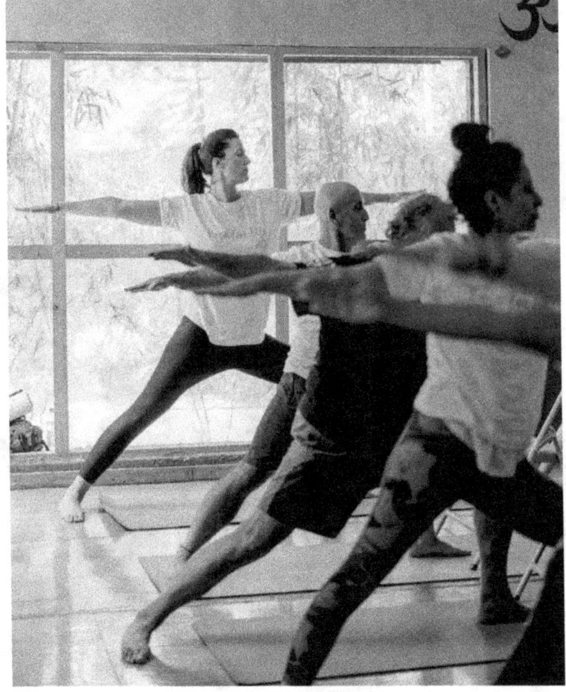

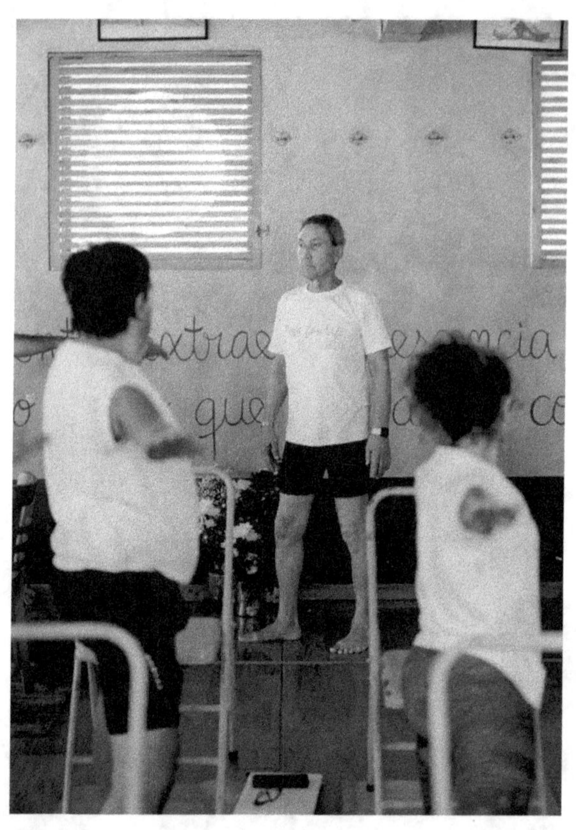

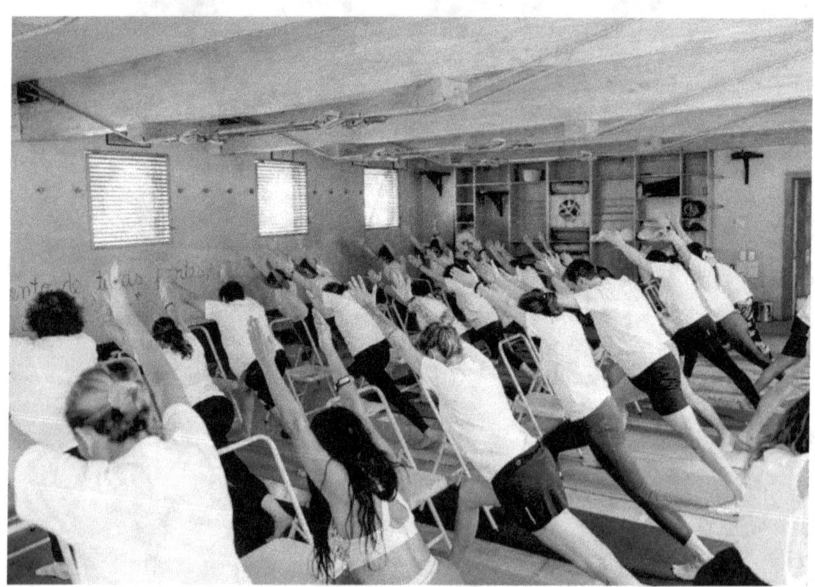

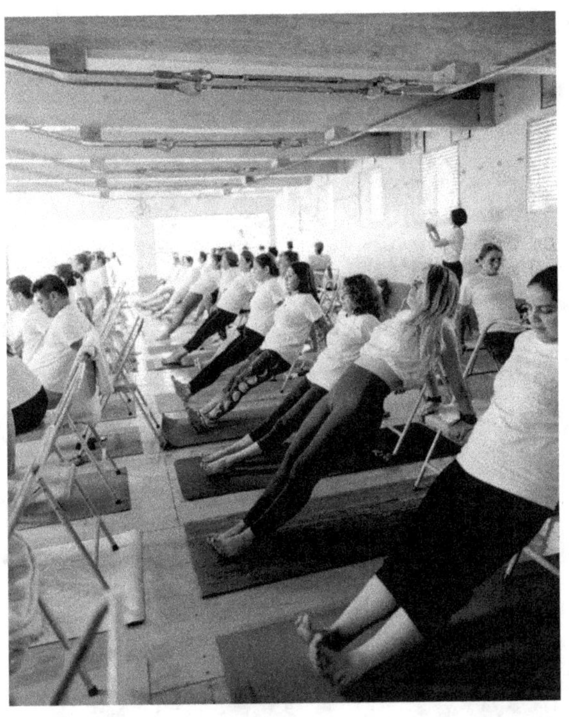

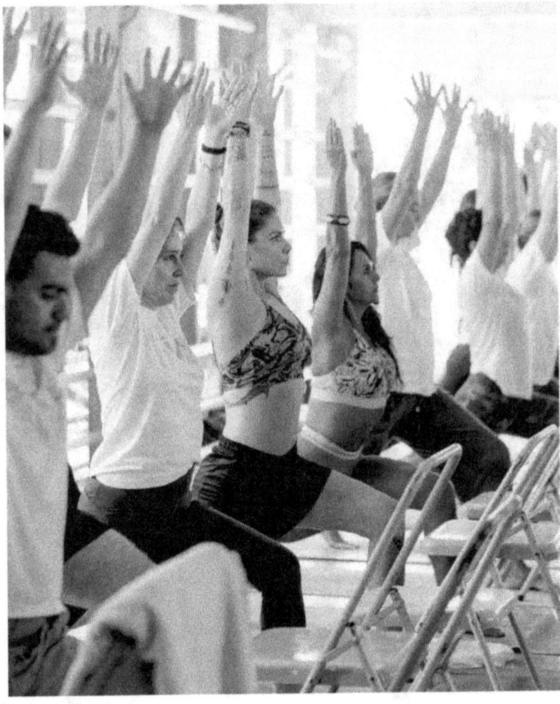

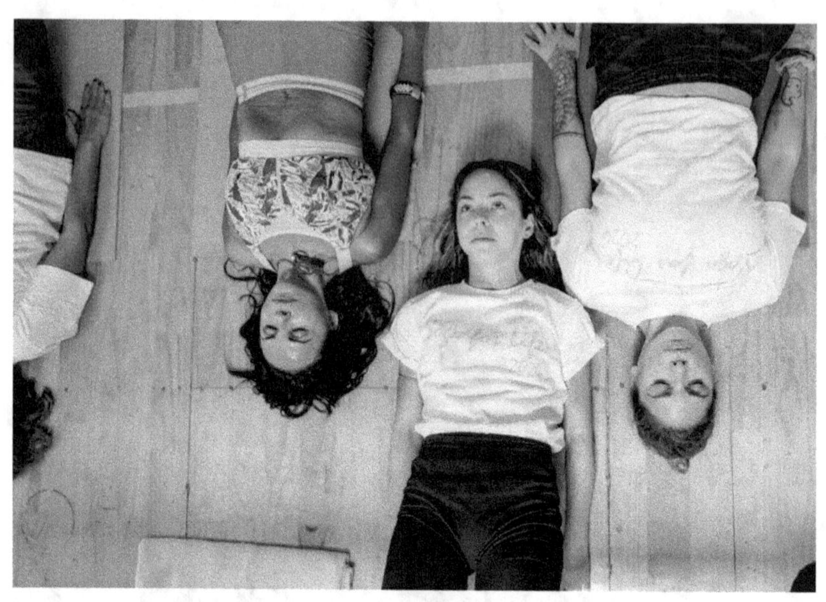

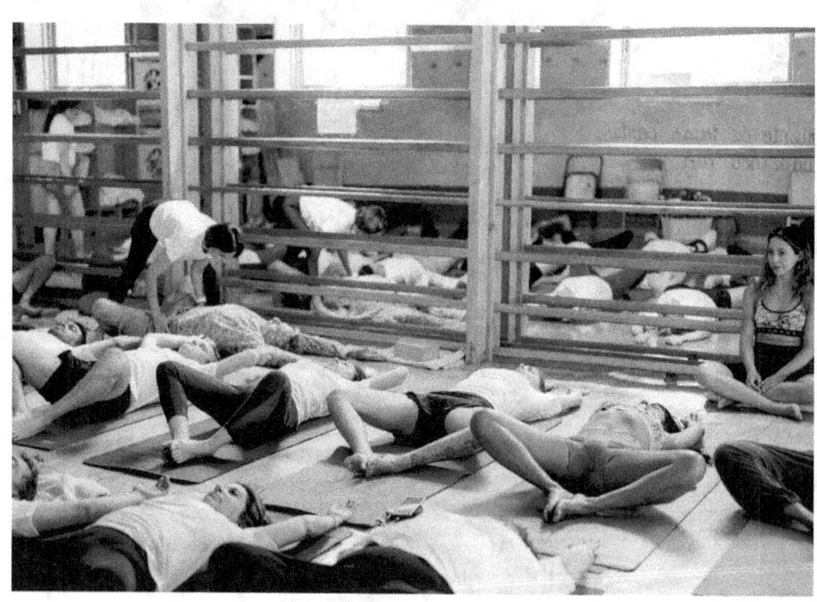

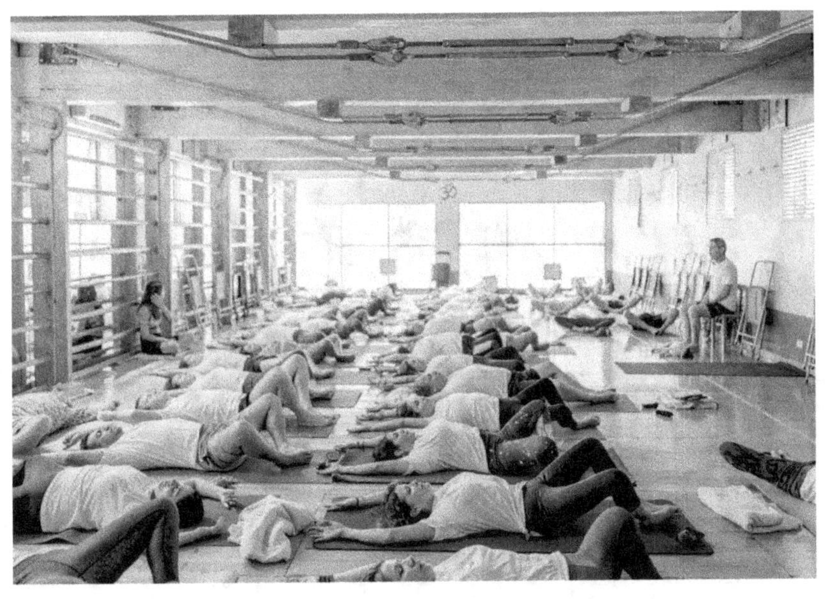

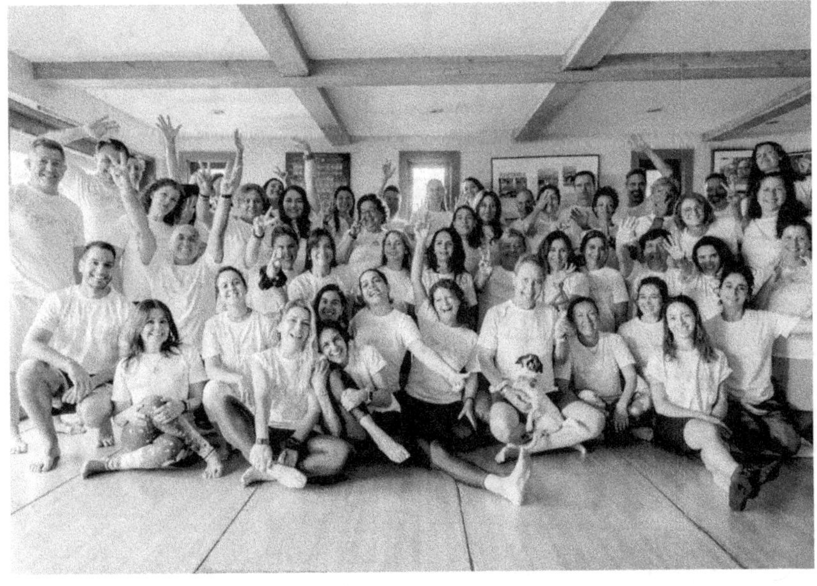

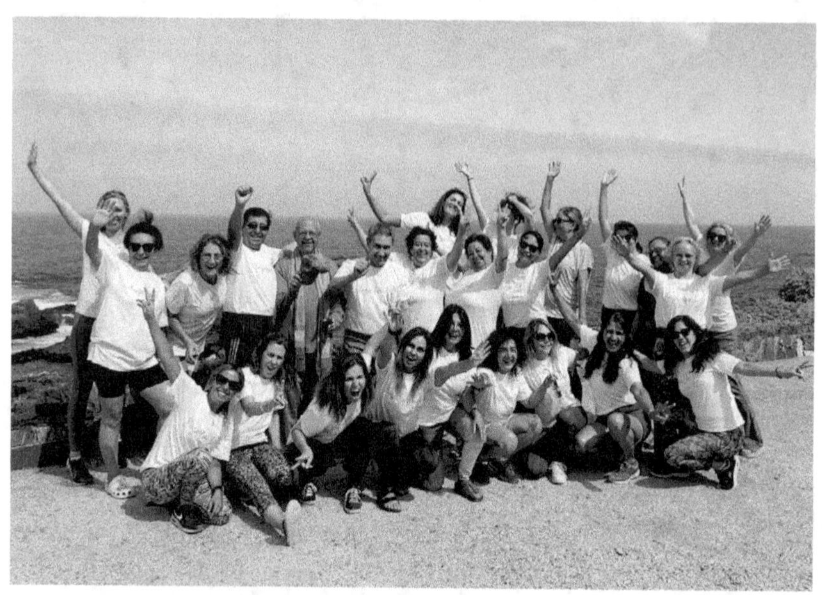

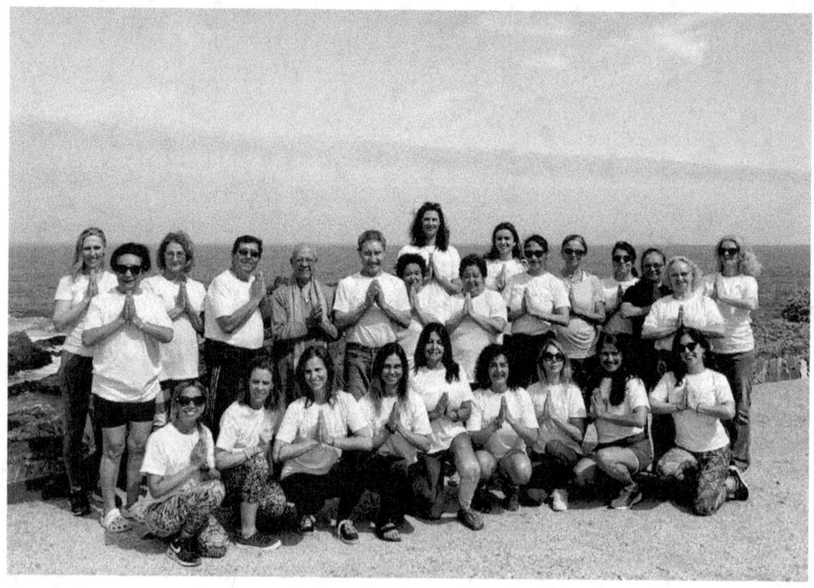

"The Yoga for Life retreat took place at
Canal Om Wellness Center
from the 1st to the 4th of February, 2024.
The teachers were Dr. Rodrigo Alcazar,
Swami Ekananda, and Gustavo Ponce".